PLANT-BASED PROSTATE CANCER DIET COOKBOOK

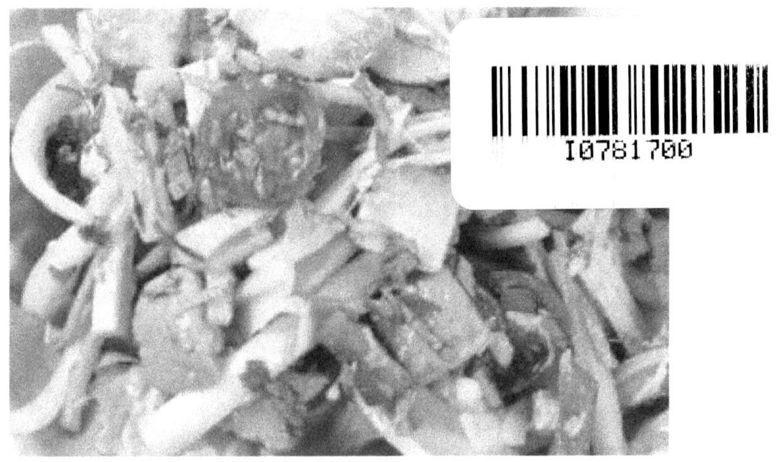

Delicious and Nourishing Plant-Based Anti-prostate Cancer Recipes for beginners

MAYER CLINTON JOSE

For further information or assistance, feel free to reach out to me at:

meyerclintonjose@gmail.com

Thank you for purchasing this book

SCAN TO SEE MORE OF MY BOOKS

TABLE OF CONTENT

INTRODUCTION

Welcome to the amazing world of the "Plant-Based Prostate Cancer Diet Cookbook," where the goodness of plants meets the hope for healing through a balanced diet. In this book, I will share my inspiring story, a true testament to the transformative nature of food.

My life changed in a big way when I got diagnosed with prostate cancer. Determined to regain my health, I searched high and low for a solution that would truly help. After digging and trying different things, I learned the power of eating mostly plants. It was like a light in the dark, bringing me back to life one meal at a time. I was amazed at the difference it made.

And now, I want to share this journey with you. The "Plant-Based Prostate Cancer Diet Cookbook" is your guide, filled with tasty recipes for your prostate and taste buds. Let these flavors surprise and delight you while the goodness of plants works its magic on your body.

Together, let's explore a world of delicious meals and better health. Join me on this journey with the "Plant-Based Prostate Cancer Diet Cookbook." We're in this together.

Benefits of Plant-Based Diets to Prostate Cancer

Decreased Risk of Advanced Prostate Cancer: Research suggests that individuals with early-stage prostate cancer who switch to a plant-based diet can significantly reduce their risk of developing advanced prostate cancer.

You create an environment that supports overall health by embracing foods primarily derived from plants such as fruits, vegetables, nuts, seeds, whole grains, and legumes. Some people even choose a strict vegan diet, abstaining entirely from animal products, while others opt for a mostly plant-based approach that includes small amounts of animal products.

Reduced Progression Risk of Diseases: A large U.S. study found that men following a vegan or strictly plant-based diet were 35% less likely to develop prostate cancer overall.

Specifically, those who adhered to a strict vegan diet experienced these improved outcomes. Additionally, plant-based diets have been associated with lower levels of prostate-specific antigen (PSA), which can help men diagnosed with low-risk or early-stage prostate cancer avoid aggressive treatments.

Enhanced Overall Health and Quality of Life: Plant-based diets offer anti-inflammatory and antioxidant effects, supporting the overall well-being of individuals with prostate cancer. Moreover, these diets are cost-effective and can help manage comorbidities like diabetes, coronary artery disease, and hypertension1. Recent research also highlights that plant-based diets can ease side effects from prostate cancer treatment, including erectile dysfunction and urinary problems while promoting better hormonal health.

A plant-based diet reduces the risk of prostate cancer and contributes to better disease management and overall health. By embracing the power of plants, you're positively impacting your well-being and potentially enhancing your quality of life.

Prostate Cancer Plant-Based Fighting Foods

Several plant-based foods are good for reducing prostate cancer risk. Here are some of them:

Cruciferous vegetables: Cruciferous vegetables like broccoli, cauliflower, kale, Brussels sprouts, and cabbage. These vegetables are rich in sulforaphane, a compound that has anticancer properties.

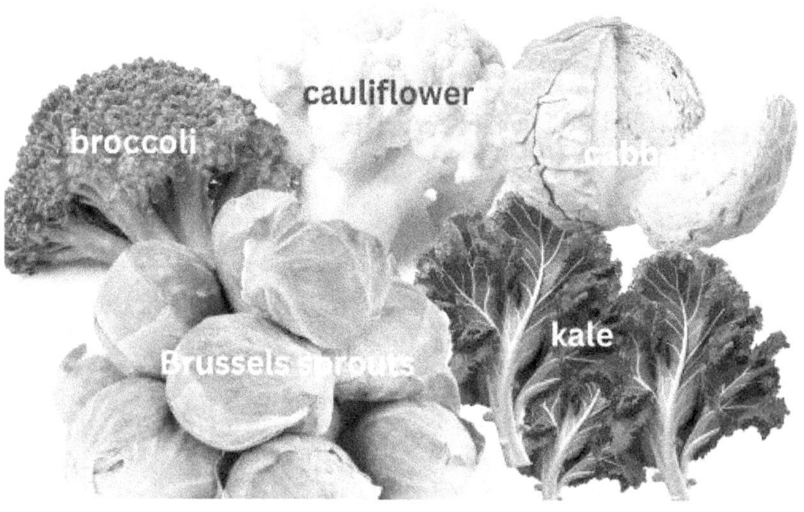

Allium vegetables: Onions and garlic fall into this category. They contain organosulfur compounds that have been found to inhibit the growth of certain types of cancer, including prostate cancer.

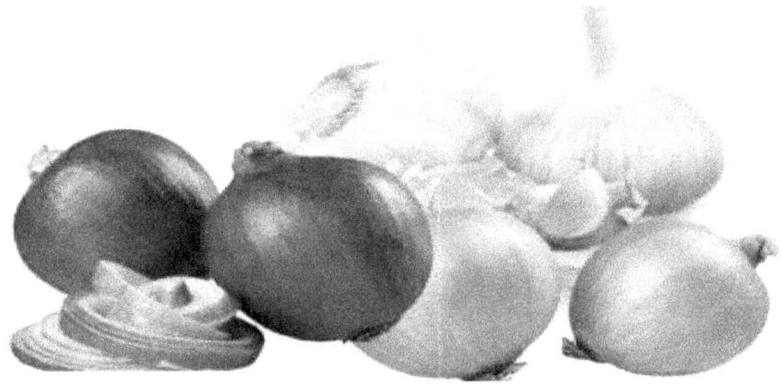

Tomatoes contain lycopene, a potent antioxidant associated with lowering the risk of prostate cancer. This antioxidant helps neutralize harmful free radicals in the body, potentially reducing cell damage and decreasing the likelihood of cancer development.

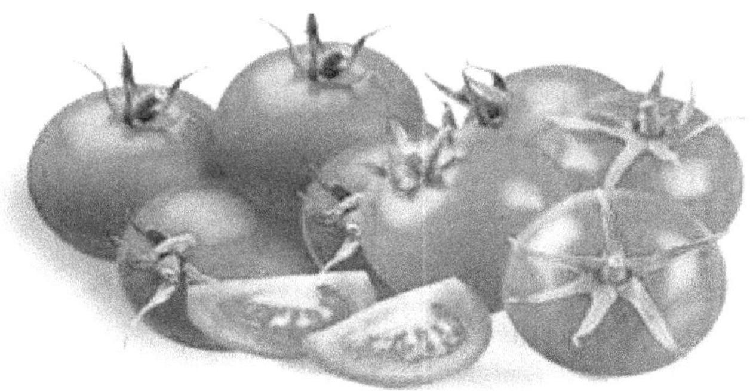

Whole grains: Whole grains are a good source of fiber, which has been associated with a lower risk of various types of cancer, including prostate cancer.

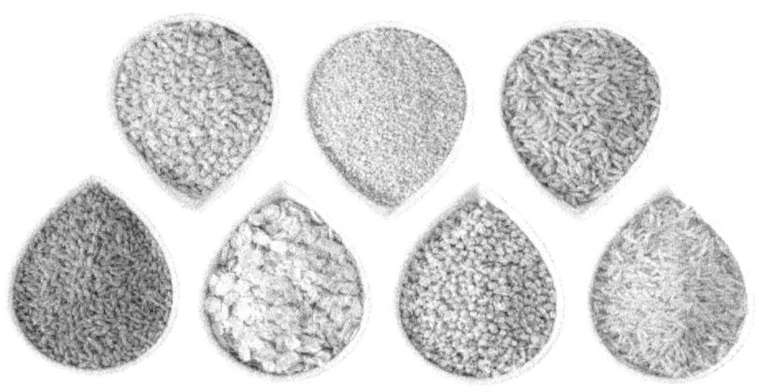

Green tea: Green tea contains polyphenols, which have been shown to inhibit the growth of cancer cells and reduce tumor growth.

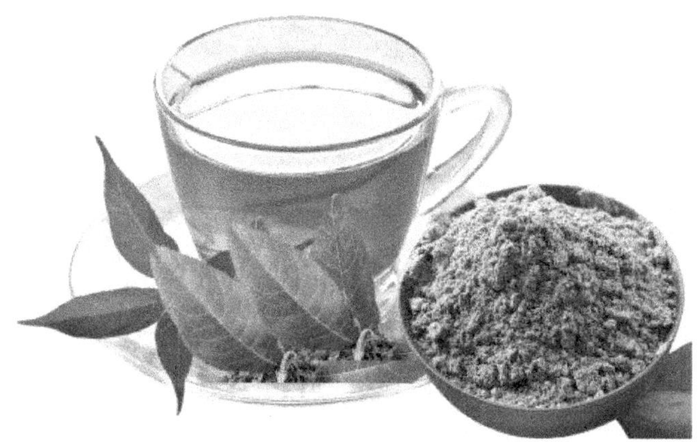

Carrots: Carrots are abundant in beta-carotene, another antioxidant with potential cancer-fighting properties. Beta-carotene safeguards cell membranes from toxins and supports the body's immune system in combating cancerous cell growth. Regular consumption of carrots may contribute to overall health and possibly aid in cancer prevention efforts.

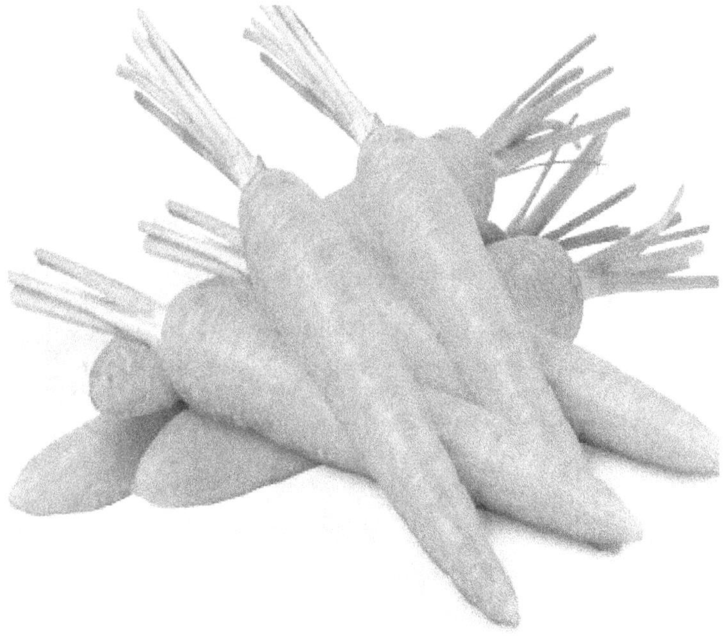

Beans: Beans are a powerful weapon against prostate cancer, rich in nutrients that promote prostate health.

The fiber content in beans aids digestion and regulates blood sugar levels, lowering cancer risk. Antioxidants like flavonoids and polyphenols in beans fight inflammation and oxidative stress, key factors in cancer progression. As a prime source of plant-based protein, beans provide a healthy alternative to red and processed meats, reducing the risk of prostate cancer. Adding beans to your diet boosts overall health and bolsters the body's defense against prostate cancer.

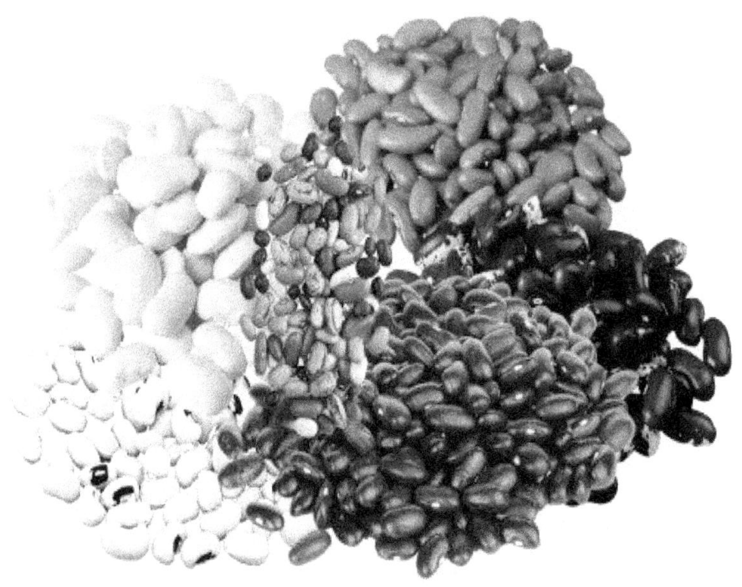

CHAPTER 1

Breakfast Recipes

Start your day right and prioritize your health with delicious breakfast recipes to fight prostate cancer. Yes, it's essential to kickstart your day with these nutrient-packed morning meals. They provide energy and give your body the essential nutrients needed to fight prostate cancer.

Scrambled Turmeric Tofu with Greens

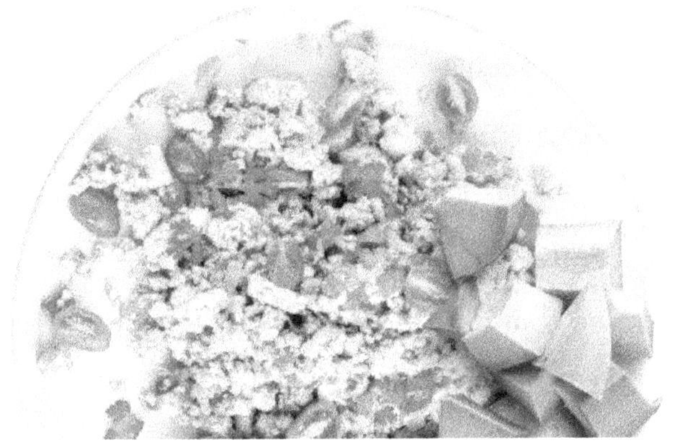

Ingredients:

- 1 block of extra firm tofu (14 ounces)
- 2 tablespoons of nutritional yeast
- 2 teaspoons of turmeric

- ½ teaspoon of smoked paprika

- ¼ teaspoon of black pepper

- Pinch of sea salt (optional)

- 2 tablespoons of plain, unsweetened plant-based milk (like oat, soy, or almond milk)

- 1 tablespoon of extra virgin olive oil

- 2 green onions, chopped

- 2 cloves of garlic, minced

- 6 ounces of sliced mushrooms

- 2 cups of chopped greens (like mustard, collard, spinach, or kale)

- ¼ cup of chopped sun-dried tomatoes

Instructions:

1. Take the tofu out of the package and wrap it in paper towels. Place it between two plates with something heavy on top for 5 minutes to drain excess liquid. You can also use a tofu press.

2. Crumble the pressed tofu into a bowl with your hands.

3. Mix in the nutritional yeast, turmeric, smoked paprika, black pepper, salt (if using), and plant-based milk.

4. Heat olive oil in a skillet over medium heat.

5. Sauté the green onions, garlic, and mushrooms in the skillet for about 5 minutes.

6. Add the crumbled tofu, chopped greens, and sun-dried tomatoes to the skillet. Sauté until the greens start to wilt, about 2 minutes.

7. Serve immediately. You can also serve with sliced avocados if you like.

Cooking Time: About 15 minutes.

Oatmeal with Fresh Fruit

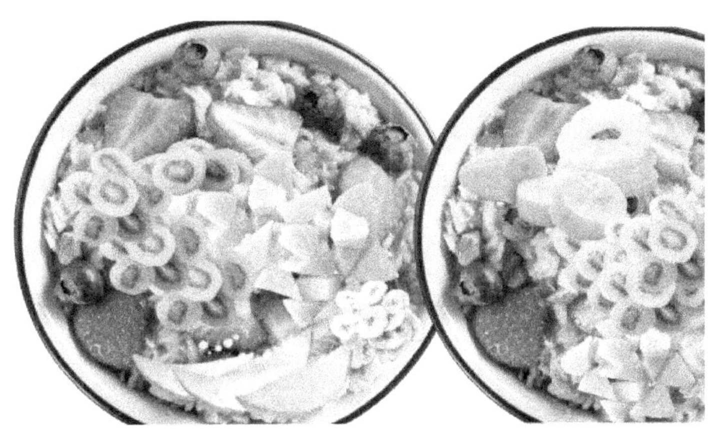

Ingredients:

- 1 cup of rolled oats
- 1 cup of plant-based milk like coconut milk or almond milk

- Natural sweeteners, like stevia (to taste)
- 1 banana, sliced
- 1/2 mango, sliced
- 1 kiwi, sliced
- 1/4 cup of diced pineapple
- 1 tablespoon of coconut flakes
- 2 tablespoons of raspberries
- Optional: Mint sprigs for garnish

Instructions:

1. Cook the rolled oats according to the package instructions.
2. Stir in the plant-based milk and sweetener, then divide the oatmeal into two bowls.
3. Arrange the sliced fruits on top of the oatmeal and sprinkle with coconut flakes.
4. Optionally, garnish with mint sprigs.
5. Serve and enjoy your delicious and nutritious breakfast!

Cooking Time: About 20 minutes.

Spinach Oat Smoothie

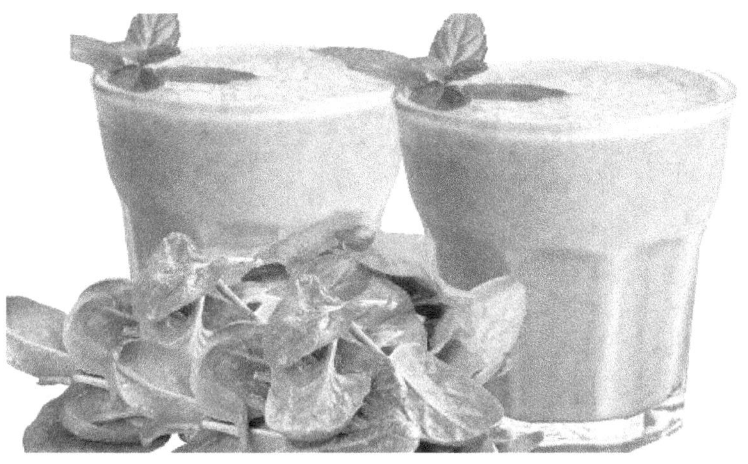

Ingredients:

- Handful of spinach
- 1 ripe banana
- 1 cup of rolled oats
- 1 cup of plant-based milk (e.g., almond milk)
- 1 tablespoon of nut butter (e.g., almond or peanut butter)

Instructions:

1. Blend all ingredients until smooth.
2. Adjust consistency by adding more milk if needed.

Total Time: About 5 minutes.

Refreshing Carrot and Celery Juice

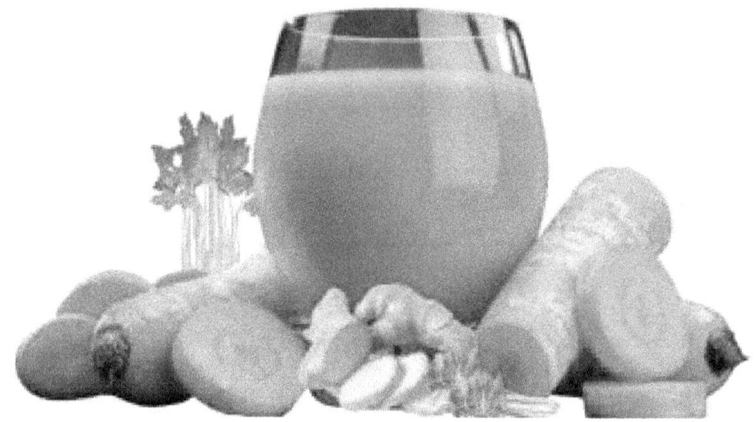

Ingredients:

- 3 large carrots
- 2 celery stalks
- 1-inch piece of fresh ginger
- Ice (optional)

Instructions:

1. Wash the carrots, celery, and ginger thoroughly.
2. Cut the carrots and celery into smaller pieces, making it easier to juice.
3. Peel the ginger and slice it into smaller chunks.

4. Add the carrots, celery, and ginger in a juicer, alternating between the ingredients to ensure even juicing.
5. Turn on the juicer and process the ingredients until you have a smooth, vibrant juice.
6. Once juiced, pour the mixture into a glass.
7. Add ice if you like and serve immediately to enjoy its fresh flavor and maximum nutritional benefits.

Total Time: About 5 minutes.

Avocado Toast with Tomato and Sprouts

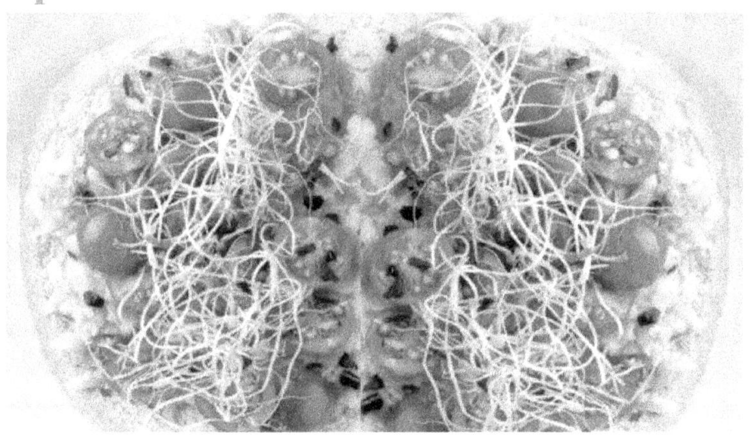

Ingredients:

- 1 ripe avocado
- 2 slices of whole-grain bread
- 2 large tomatoes

- Alfalfa sprouts or microgreens
- Lemon juice
- Salt
- Pepper

Instructions:

1. Peel and pit the avocado. Scoop out the flesh into a bowl.

2. Add a squeeze of lemon juice, a pinch of salt, and a dash of pepper to the avocado.

3. Mash the avocado mixture with a fork until smooth and well combined.

4. Toast the whole-grain bread slices until golden brown and crispy.

5. Slice the tomato into thin rounds.

6. Once the toast is ready, spread the mashed avocado evenly over each slice.

7. Arrange the tomato slices on top of the avocado spread.

8. Sprinkle a handful of alfalfa sprouts or microgreens over the tomatoes.

9. For extra zest, drizzle a little more lemon juice over the top.

10. Serve immediately and enjoy the delicious and nutritious avocado toast!

Total Time: 10 minutes.

Turmeric Overnight Oats

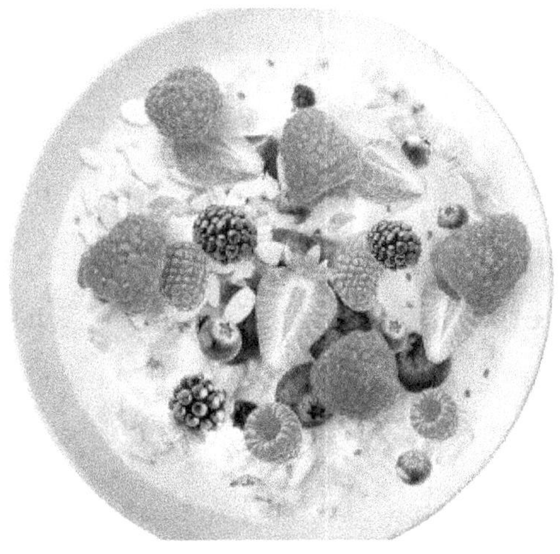

Ingredients:

- 1 cup of rolled oats
- One cup of any plant-based milk (like unsweetened almond milk)
- 1 teaspoon of ground turmeric
- 1 tablespoon of chia seeds
- 1 ripe banana, mashed

- Optional toppings: sliced almonds, berries, or a drizzle of maple syrup

Instructions:

1. Combine the rolled oats, almond milk, ground turmeric, chia seeds, and mashed banana in a jar or bowl.
2. Combine all the ingredients until they are thoroughly mixed.
3. Cover the jar or bowl and refrigerate overnight for at least 6 hours.
4. In the morning, stir the mixture well. Add the additional almond milk to achieve your desired consistency, and stir well.
5. Add optional toppings like sliced almonds, berries, or a drizzle of maple syrup if desired.
6. Enjoy your delicious and nutritious vegan turmeric overnight oats!

Prep Time: 10 min, Rest Time: 8 hours

Total Time: 8 hours 10 mins

CHAPTER 2

Lunch Recipes

Elevate your midday with tantalizing recipes specifically crafted to fight prostate cancer. These Recipes satisfy your taste buds and nourish your body with essential nutrients. With each bite, you're not just enjoying a delicious meal but also taking a proactive step towards a healthier, prostate cancer-resistant lifestyle.

Broccoli, Garlic, and Lemon Penne

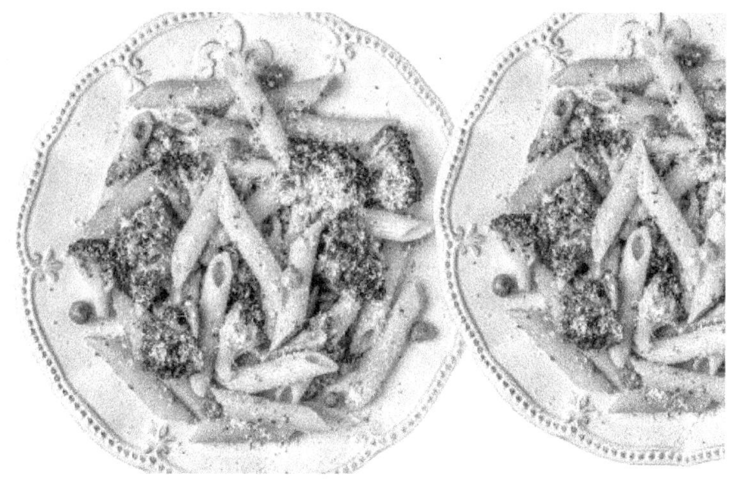

Ingredients:

- Whole wheat penne pasta

- Broccoli florets

- Garlic cloves

- Lemon zest and juice

- Olive oil

- Salt and pepper

Instructions:

1. Prepare the penne pasta as directed on the package.

2. In a separate pan, sauté minced garlic in olive oil until it smells good.

3. Add broccoli florets and cook until they're just tender.

4. Mix the cooked penne with the broccoli, garlic, lemon zest, and lemon juice.

5. Season with salt and pepper.

Prep time: 15 minutes or less

Total time: 30 minutes or less

Grapefruit, Avocado, and Baby Greens Crab Salad

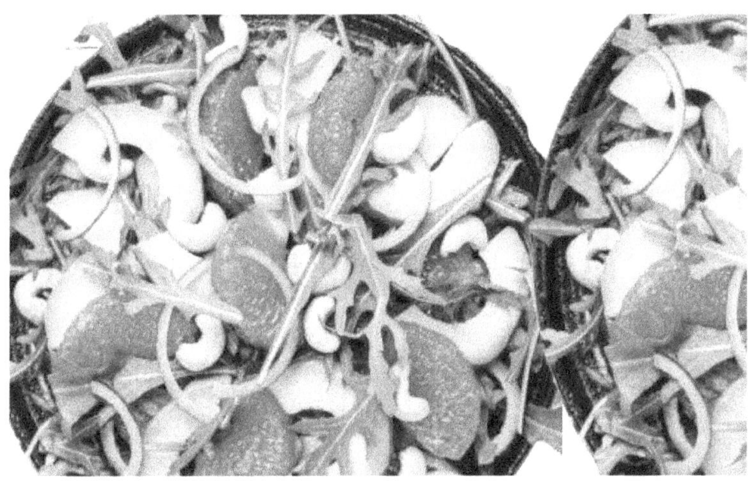

Ingredients:

- 1 pink or ruby red grapefruit
- 2 tablespoons of extra-virgin olive oil
- 1 tablespoon of fresh lemon juice
- 1/2-pound of fresh crabmeat, picked over for cartilage
- 2 tablespoons of chopped fresh Italian parsley
- 1 tablespoon of chopped fresh chives, plus more for garnishing
- 1/4 teaspoon of granulated sugar

- Salt and freshly ground black pepper

- 1/2 avocado, sliced

- 4 cups of (or 6.5-ounce bag) cut baby Bibb or Boston lettuce

Instructions:

1. Peel and segment the grapefruit over a bowl to catch the juice. Set aside 1 tablespoon of juice and the grapefruit pieces separately.

2. Whisk together the olive oil, lemon juice, sugar, and the reserved grapefruit juice in a small bowl to make the dressing.

3. Combine the crabmeat, chopped parsley, and chopped chives in another bowl. Add 1 1/2 tablespoons of the prepared dressing and toss gently to combine—season with salt and pepper to taste.

4. Toss the lettuce with the remaining dressing until evenly coated. Divide the dressed lettuce onto individual plates.

5. Top each plate of lettuce with a scoop of the crabmeat salad.

6. Arrange the reserved grapefruit segments and avocado slices around the crabmeat salad.

7. Garnish with additional chopped chives if desired.

8. Serve salad immediately, and enjoy!

Total time: 30 minutes or less

Rice Noodles with Shrimp, Bok Choy, and Mint

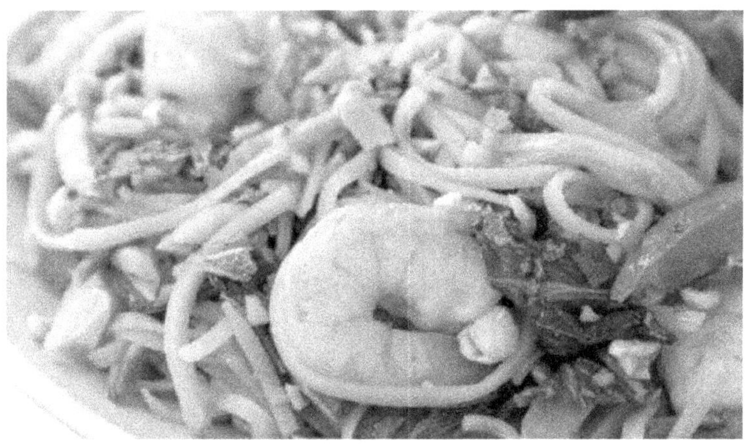

Ingredients:

- 6 ounces of thin rice noodles
- 1/4 cup of reduced-sodium soy sauce
- 3 tablespoons of rice vinegar

- 3 tablespoons of hoisin sauce

- 1 tablespoon of canola oil

- 2 garlic cloves, minced

- 1 small jalapeño pepper, deseeded and chopped

- 1 (2-inch) piece of peeled fresh ginger, minced

- 3/4-pound shrimp, peeled and deveined

- 2 scallions, thinly sliced (using only the white and light green parts)

- 2 carrots, shredded

- 1 red bell pepper, thinly sliced after removing the seeds

- 1 head bok choy, cored and thinly sliced

- 1 tablespoon of dark sesame oil

- 2 tablespoons of chopped fresh mint

- 2 tablespoons of chopped peanuts

Instructions:

1. Cook the rice noodles according to the package instructions. Once cooked, drain well and pat dry with paper towels.

2. Mix the soy sauce, rice vinegar, and hoisin sauce in a small bowl to make the sauce mixture.

3. Add the canola oil in a large skillet or wok over medium-high heat. Add the minced garlic, chopped jalapeño, and minced ginger. Cook for about 1 minute until fragrant.

4. Add the peeled and deveined shrimp to the skillet, along with the sliced scallions, shredded carrots, bell pepper strips, and thinly sliced bok choy. Stir-fry the mixture for 2 to 3 minutes, until the shrimp turn pink and the vegetables are tender.

5. Add the cooked rice noodles to the skillet and toss to combine with the shrimp and vegetables.

6. Pour the prepared sauce mixture over the noodle and shrimp mixture. Stir well to coat all the ingredients evenly with the sauce.

7. Transfer the stir-fried noodles and shrimp to a serving bowl.

8. Drizzle the dark sesame oil over the top of the dish.

9. Garnish with chopped fresh mint and chopped peanuts.

10. Serve immediately and enjoy!

Total time: About 35min

Asparagus, Lima Bean & Almond Pasta

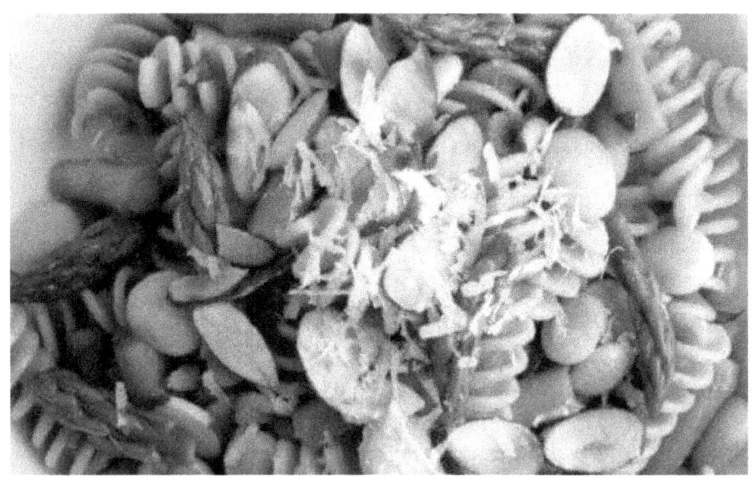

Ingredients:

- 3 tablespoons of sliced almonds
- 1 tablespoon of sea salt (for boiling pasta)
- 8 ounces of whole wheat rotini or penne pasta
- 1 pound of green asparagus, trimmed and cut into 1-inch pieces
- 1 cup of frozen baby lima beans
- 3 tablespoons of olive oil
- 2 cloves of garlic, thinly sliced

- 1 dried pepper pod, deseeded (optional)
- 3 tablespoons of chopped Italian parsley
- 1 tablespoon of grated Parmigiano Reggiano cheese (optional)
- Sea salt and black pepper to taste

Instructions:

1. In a heavy-bottomed pan, toast the sliced almonds over medium heat until golden. Please move it to a bowl and keep it aside.
2. Boil a large pot of water with salt. Add the pasta and cook according to package instructions, but stop cooking 3 minutes before the suggested time. Add the asparagus and frozen lima beans to the boiling pasta and continue cooking for 2 more minutes. Reserve 1 cup of pasta water, then drain the pasta and vegetables, ensuring they are slightly undercooked.
3. In a deep pan or wok, heat olive oil over medium-high heat. Once the oil is hot, add the thinly sliced garlic and dried pepper pod (if using). Cook the garlic until it turns light golden, which should take around 3 minutes. Be careful not to burn the garlic.

4. Add the chopped parsley to the pan and stir-fry for 1 minute. Pour 1/4 cup of the reserved pasta water into the pan and bring to a simmer.

5. Add the toasted almonds to the pan and reduce the heat to medium. If the pan becomes dry, gradually add more pasta water as needed.

6. Add the drained pasta, asparagus, and lima beans to the pan. Stir well to combine, then gradually add the remaining pasta water, stirring continuously as it reduces.

7. Sprinkle the grated Parmigiano Reggiano cheese over the pasta mixture and season with black pepper to taste. Mix everything well and let it cook for another minute.

8. Taste for seasoning and adjust with additional salt and pepper if needed.

9. Serve the asparagus, lima bean, and almond pasta immediately, and enjoy its delicious flavors!

Prep Tim: 10 min

Total time: 30 min

Green Tea Smoothie

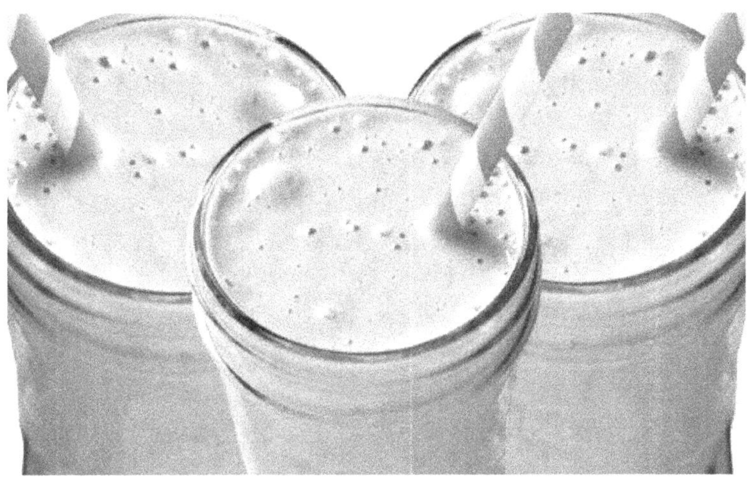

Ingredients:

- 3/4 cup of cooled green tea

- 1 frozen banana

- 1/4 cup of fresh or frozen pineapple or mango

- 1 cup of tightly packed baby spinach or kale leaves

- 1 tablespoon of well-stirred almond butter

- 1 tablespoon of ground flaxseed

- 1 tablespoon of hemp seeds

- 1/4 teaspoon of cinnamon

Instructions:

1. In a blender, add all ingredients in the order listed.
2. Blend until smooth, adjusting the consistency by adding more green tea if needed.
3. Once smooth, pour into a glass and enjoy your nutritious green tea smoothie!

Total time: 5min

Lentil and Vegetable Stir-Fry

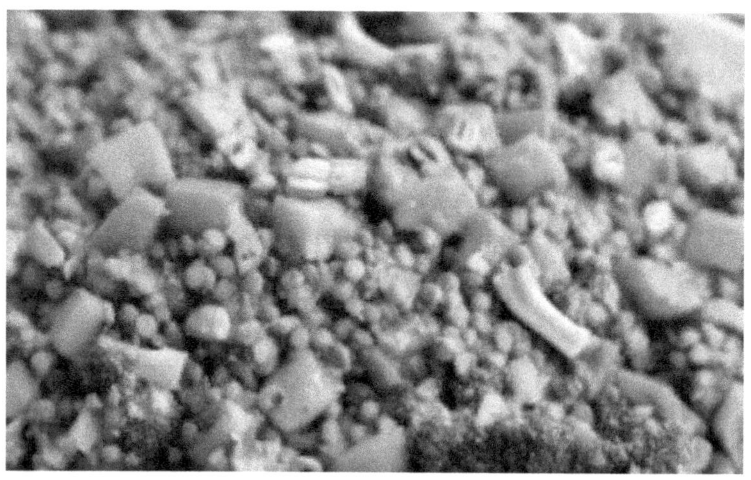

Ingredients:

- 1 cup of dried green lentils, rinsed
- 2 cups of water

- 1 tablespoon of olive oil

- 1 onion, chopped

- 2 cloves of garlic, minced

- 1 bell pepper, diced

- 2 carrots, sliced

- 1 zucchini, diced

- 1 cup of broccoli florets

- 1 tablespoon of low-sodium soy sauce

- 1 tablespoon of balsamic vinegar

- 1 teaspoon of dried thyme

- Salt and pepper to taste

- Cooked brown rice or quinoa for serving (optional)

Instruction:

1. Place the rinsed lentils and water in a medium saucepan. Bring the mixture to a boil, then reduce the heat to low and let it simmer for 20-25 minutes until the lentils are tender. Once cooked, drain any excess water and set the lentils aside.

2. In a large skillet or wok, heat olive oil over medium heat. Add chopped onion and minced garlic, and sauté until fragrant, about 2 minutes.

3. Add diced bell pepper, sliced carrots, diced zucchini, and broccoli florets to the skillet. Cook the vegetables for 5-7 minutes, stirring occasionally, until they become tender.

4. Stir in the cooked lentils, low-sodium soy sauce, balsamic vinegar, and dried thyme. Cook for an additional 2-3 minutes to heat through and allow flavors to blend.

5. Season with salt and pepper according to your taste preferences.

6. If desired, serve the lentil and vegetable stir-fry with cooked brown rice or quinoa. Enjoy your nutritious and flavorful plant-based lunch!

Cook Time: Approximately 30 minutes

Chickpea Salad with Avocado Dressing

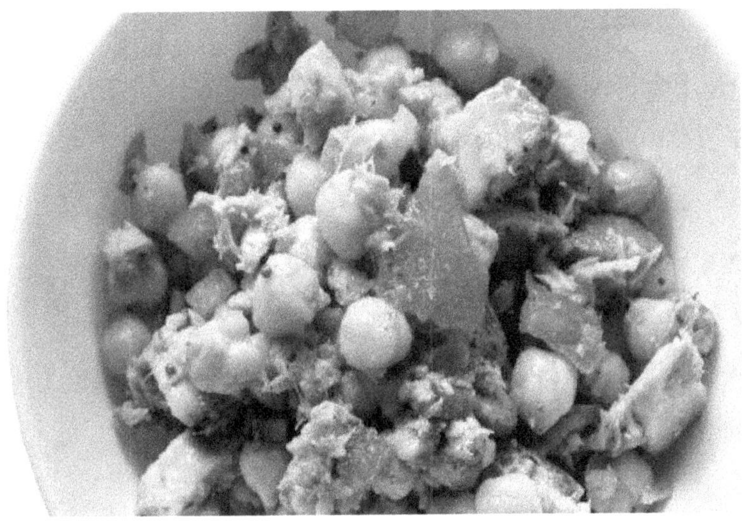

Ingredients:

For the Salad:

- 2 cans of (15 ounces each) chickpeas, drained and rinsed
- 1 cucumber, diced
- 1 red bell pepper, diced
- 1 cup of cherry tomatoes, halved
- 1/4 cup of red onion, finely chopped

- 1/4 cup of fresh parsley, chopped

For the Avocado Dressing:

- 1 ripe avocado, peeled and pitted
- 1/4 cup of fresh lemon juice
- 2 tablespoons of olive oil
- 1 clove of garlic, minced
- 1 teaspoon of Dijon mustard
- Salt and pepper to taste
- Water, as needed, to thin the dressing

Preparation:

1. Combine the drained and rinsed chickpeas, diced cucumber, red bell pepper, halved cherry tomatoes, finely chopped red onion, and chopped fresh parsley in a large mixing bowl. Set aside.
2. Mix the peeled and pitted avocado, fresh lemon juice, olive oil, minced garlic, Dijon mustard, salt, and pepper in a blender or food processor.
3. Blend until smooth, adding water as needed to achieve your desired consistency for the dressing.

4. Pour the avocado dressing over the chickpea salad ingredients in the mixing bowl.

5. Gently toss until the salad is evenly coated with the dressing.

6. Taste and adjust seasoning if necessary.

7. Serve the chickpea salad immediately or chill in the refrigerator for 30 minutes before serving to allow the flavors to meld. Enjoy your vibrant and satisfying plant-based lunch!

Cook Time: Approximately 15 minutes

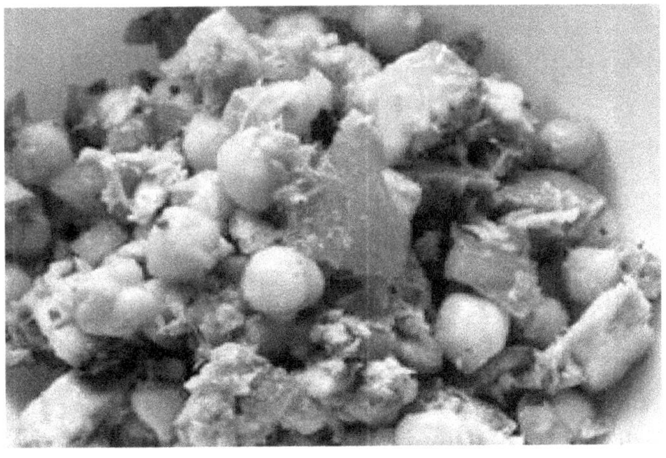

Dinner Recipes

Fight prostate cancer with plant-based anti-prostate cancer dinner recipes. Each meal is a delicious defense against illness. Together, let's make a change—one plate at a time.

Black Bean Curry

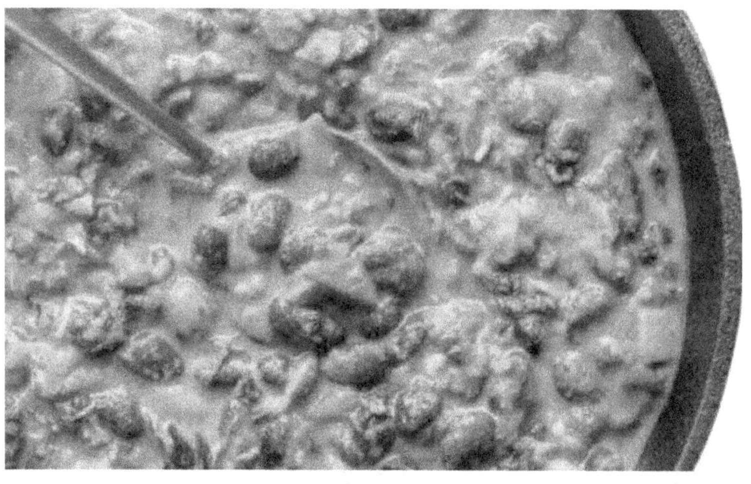

Ingredients:

- 3 tablespoons of plant-based spread
- 1 teaspoon of cumin seeds
- 1 large onion, finely chopped

- 4 large garlic cloves, crushed

- 5 medium tomatoes, weighing about 350 grams, seeded and finely chopped.

- ¼ teaspoon of cayenne pepper (optional)

- ½ tablespoon of ground coriander

- ½ teaspoon of garam masala

- ½ teaspoon of turmeric

- cups of cooked black beans (roughly two cans)

- 2 - 2.5 cups of vegetable stock

- Salt to taste

- 4 tablespoons of coconut cream

- 3 tablespoons of fresh cilantro leaves, finely chopped (optional)

- 1.5 teaspoons of kasuri methi (optional but recommended)

Instructions:

1. Melt the plant-based spread in a pan over medium-high heat. Add the cumin seeds.

2. Add the chopped onion once the cumin seeds brown and crackle (after about two minutes). Cook for about five minutes until the onions are lightly browned.

3. Add the crushed garlic and cook for one more minute.

4. Stir in the chopped tomatoes, reduce the heat to medium, and cook for about five to six minutes, stirring often, until the tomatoes are soft and disintegrating.

5. Add the optional cayenne pepper, ground coriander, garam masala, and turmeric. Stir thoroughly and let it cook for an additional minute.

6. Add the drained and rinsed black beans and vegetable stock. Season with salt to taste (about ¼ teaspoon; adjust according to the saltiness of your vegetable stock).

7. Increase the heat to high until the mixture is simmering lively, then reduce to medium and simmer for about twelve minutes until the curry thickens to your liking.

8. Stir in the coconut cream, half of the chopped cilantro leaves, and the kasuri methi (crumbled between your fingers). Mix well.

9. Sprinkle the remaining cilantro leaves on top before serving.

10. Enjoy this flavorful and comforting black bean curry with cooked brown rice or whole wheat bread!

Cook Time: 31 Minutes

Quinoa Stuffed Bell Peppers

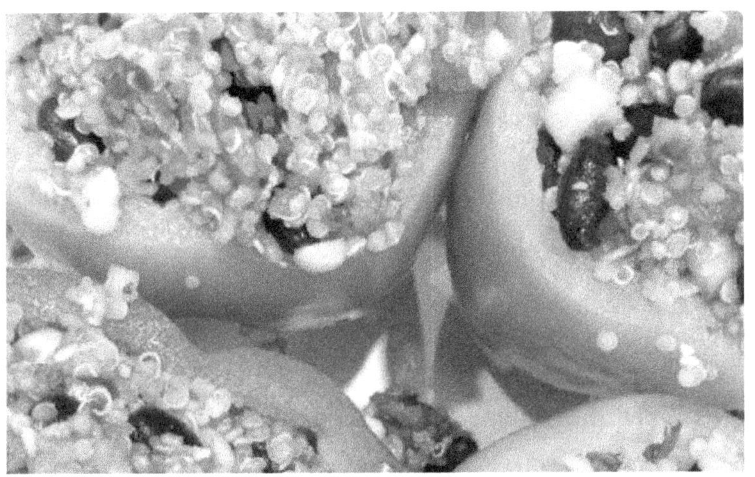

Ingredients:

- 1 cup of quinoa
- 2 cups of water
- 4 bell peppers
- 1 can of black beans (Cooked)
- 1 cup of corn
- 1 onion
- 2 cloves of garlic
- 1 teaspoon of cumin
- 1 teaspoon of chili powder
- Salt and pepper to taste

Instructions:

1. Rinse the quinoa under cold water in a fine-mesh strainer.

2. In a saucepan, combine the rinsed quinoa and water. Bring to a boil, then reduce the heat to low, cover, and simmer for about 15 minutes, or until the quinoa is fluffy and the water is absorbed. Take it off the heat and allow it to rest, covered, for 5 minutes.

3. While the quinoa is cooking, preheat your oven to 375°F (190°C).

4. Meanwhile, prepare the bell peppers by cutting off the tops and removing the seeds and membranes.

5. Finely chop the onion and mince the garlic cloves.

6. In a skillet, heat a bit of oil over medium heat. Add the chopped onion and minced garlic, and cook until softened, for about 5 minutes.

7. Drain and rinse the black beans and corn. Add them to the skillet along with the onions and garlic.

8. Season the mixture with cumin, chili powder, salt, and pepper. Stir well to combine.

9. Once the quinoa is cooked, add it to the skillet with the bean and corn mixture. Stir until everything is evenly combined.

10. Stuff each bell pepper with the quinoa mixture, pressing down gently to pack it in.

11. Place the stuffed bell peppers in a baking dish and cover with aluminum foil.

12. Bake in the preheated oven for about 30 minutes or until the peppers are tender.

13. Remove the foil and bake for another 5 minutes to lightly brown the tops of the peppers.

14. Serve the quinoa stuffed bell peppers hot, garnished with fresh herbs if desired. Enjoy this wholesome and flavorful meal!

Cooking Time: About 45 minutes

Stir-fried kale and Broccoli Florets

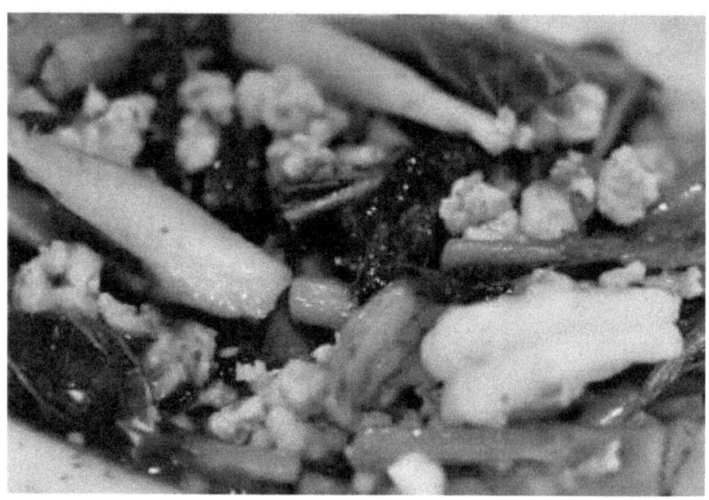

Ingredients:

- 1/8 cup of extra virgin olive oil

- 7 cloves of garlic, sliced

- 1 chile of pepper, chopped (optional)

- 1 head of fresh broccoli, chopped

- 1 bunch of kale, stems removed and chopped

- 1/4 cup of sun-dried tomatoes, cut into thin strips

- Juice of 2 limes

- Salt to taste

Instructions:

1. Heat the extra virgin olive oil in a large wok or skillet over high heat.
2. Add the sliced garlic and chopped chile pepper (if using). Cook and stir for about 2 minutes, stirring frequently until the garlic is fragrant.
3. Stir in the chopped broccoli and cook for about 1 minute.
4. Add the chopped kale to the skillet and cook for about 2 minutes, stirring frequently until the kale starts to wilt.
5. Stir in the sun-dried tomatoes and cook for another minute.
6. Pour in the juice of 2 limes and season the mixture with salt to taste. Toss everything well to combine.
7. Remove from heat once the vegetables are cooked to your liking and well coated with the lime juice and seasonings.
8. Serve and enjoy!

CookTime:10 mins

Lentil Soup

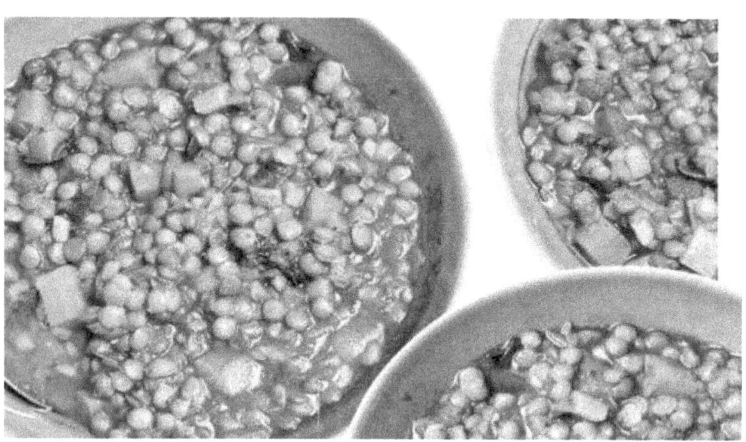

Ingredients:

- 1/4 cup of olive oil
- 1 onion, chopped
- 2 carrots, diced
- 2 stalks of celery, chopped
- 2 cloves of garlic, minced
- 1 bay leaf
- 1 teaspoon of dried oregano
- 1 teaspoon of dried basil
- 2 cups of dry lentils
- 8 cups of water
- 1 (14.5 ounces) can crushed tomatoes

- 1/2 cup of spinach, washed and thinly sliced.

- 2 tablespoons of vinegar

- Salt to taste

- Ground black pepper to taste

Instructions:

1. Heat the olive oil in a large pot on medium heat.

2. Add the chopped onions, diced carrots, and chopped celery. Cook and stir until the onion is tender, which usually takes about 3 to 5 minutes.

3. Stir in the minced garlic, bay leaf, dried oregano, and dried basil. Cook for an extra 2 minutes, stirring occasionally.

4. Add the dry lentils to the pot, then pour in the water and add the crushed tomatoes. Bring the mixture to a boil.

5. Once boiling, reduce the heat and let the soup simmer until the lentils are tender. This usually takes at least 1 hour, but you can cook it longer for a richer flavor.

6. When the lentils are cooked, stir in the thinly sliced spinach and cook until it wilts, which usually takes just a few minutes.

7. Stir in the vinegar, then season the soup with salt and pepper to taste. Taste and adjust seasoning if necessary to suit your preference.

8. Serve the hot lentil soup and enjoy its hearty and comforting flavors!

Total Cook Time: 1 hr. 35 mins

Spinach and Mushroom Pasta

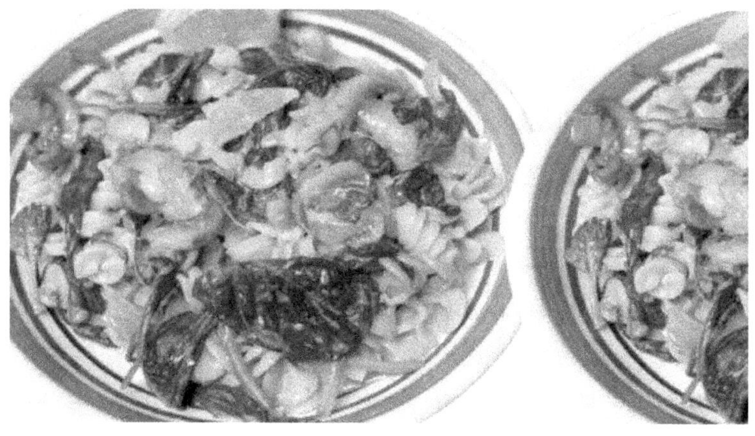

Ingredients:

- 1 tablespoon of olive oil
- 1 yellow onion, sliced
- 8 ounces of white mushrooms, sliced
- 2 cloves of garlic, minced

- 1/4 teaspoon of crushed red chile flakes

- 1 teaspoon of kosher salt

- 4 cups of vegetable broth

- 8 ounces of rotini pasta

- 1 (5 ounces) bag of baby spinach

- 1/2 cup of grated Parmesan cheese

- 1 teaspoon of lemon juice

Instructions:

1. Heat the olive oil in a large skillet over medium-high heat until it shimmers.

2. Add sliced onion and mushrooms. Cook for about 7 minutes until they're tender and golden.

3. Stir in minced garlic and crushed red chile flakes. Cook for 1 minute more.

4. Add kosher salt, vegetable broth, and rotini pasta to the skillet. Bring to a boil.

5. Reduce heat, cover the skillet, and let it simmer for 10 minutes. Stir halfway through.

6. Turn off the heat. Add the baby spinach to the skillet, cover, and let it sit for 2 minutes until it wilts.

7. Stir in grated Parmesan cheese and lemon juice.

8. Serve the mushroom spinach pasta immediately and enjoy this delicious and comforting meal!

Total Cook Time:25 mins

Chickpea Curry

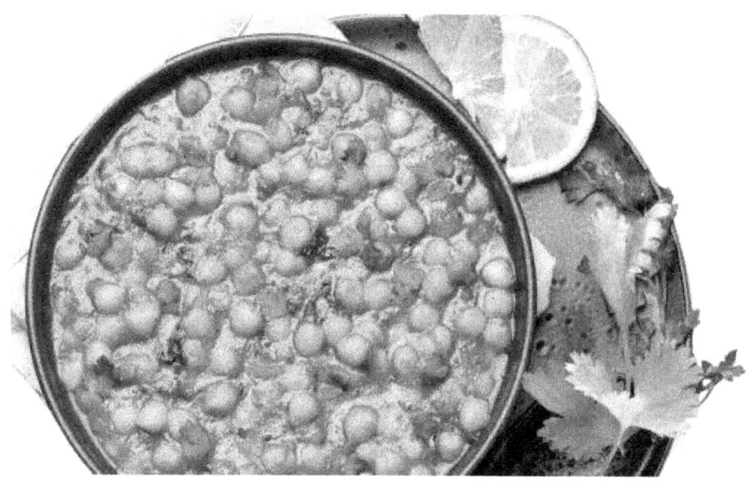

Ingredients:

- 2 tablespoons of vegetable oil or coconut oil

- 1 medium onion, sliced

- 3 cloves of garlic, minced

- 1/4 teaspoon of crushed red pepper flakes

- 1-2 tablespoons of curry powder

- 1 teaspoon of cumin

- 1 (15-ounce) can of crushed tomatoes

- 1 (13.5 ounces) can of coconut milk

- 2 (15-ounce) cans of chickpeas, drained and rinsed

- Salt and pepper, to taste

- Freshly chopped cilantro and lime wedges are used for garnish (optional).

- whole wheat bread or brown rice, to serve (optional)

Instructions:

1. Heat vegetable or coconut oil in a large, heavy-bottomed pot or high-walled pan over medium-low heat.

2. Add sliced onion, minced garlic, and crushed red pepper to the pot. Cook, stirring occasionally, until the onion is softened and deep golden, which usually takes about 15 minutes. If the onions start to dry out, add a tablespoon of water at a time.

3. Increase the heat to medium. Add curry powder and cumin to the pot and stir until toasted about 1 minute.

4. Pour in the crushed tomatoes and gently scrape the bottom of the pan with a spoon to release any browned spices or onions stuck to the bottom.

5. Add the coconut milk and drained chickpeas to the pot. Mix thoroughly and lower the heat to a simmer. Let simmer until the sauce is thickened and the chickpeas are slightly softened, which typically takes about 10 minutes, stirring occasionally.

6. Season the chickpea curry with salt and pepper to taste, and adjust other seasonings as necessary.

7. Garnish with chopped cilantro and serve with lime wedges. Enjoy your delicious chickpea curry over brown rice or with whole wheat bread.

Total Cook Time:40mins

Sweet Potato and Black Bean Taco

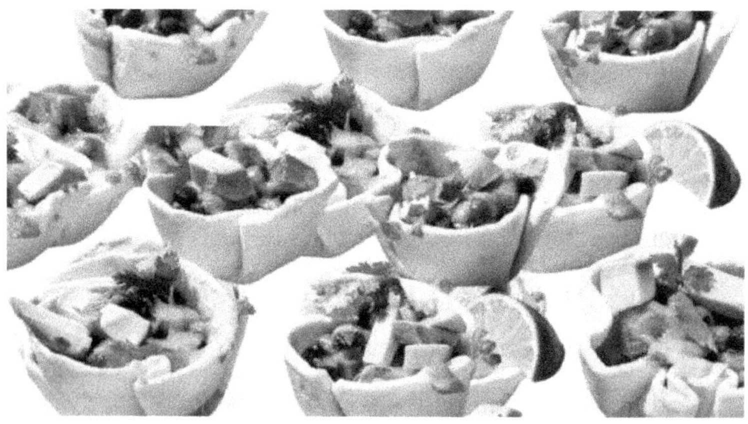

Ingredients:

- Cooking spray
- 12 (4-inch) flour tortillas
- 1 tablespoon of olive oil
- 1 cup of peeled and chopped sweet potato
- 1 yellow onion, chopped
- 1 jalapeño, seeded and minced
- 3 cloves of garlic, minced
- 1 can of undrained black beans in mild chili sauce (15 ounces).
- 1/4 teaspoon of salt
- 1/4 teaspoon of black pepper
- Mexican-style cheese blend or shredded queso quesadilla (3 ounces)
- 1 small avocado, diced
- Chopped fresh cilantro for garnish
- Lime wedges and lime crema for serving

Instructions:

1. Set the oven temperature to 350°F (175°C)—
2. coat 12 (2 1/2-inch) muffin cups with cooking spray.

3. Press 1 tortilla into the bottom of each muffin cup, pleating edges as needed to fit.

4. Warm the olive oil in a large skillet over medium-high heat.

5. Add chopped sweet potato to the skillet; cook until tender, about 10 minutes.

6. Add chopped onion to the skillet; cook until softened, for about 2 to 3 minutes.

7. Stir in minced jalapeño and minced garlic; cook until fragrant, about 2 minutes.

8. Add black beans (undrained), salt, and black pepper to the skillet; stir to combine.

9. Divide the bean mixture evenly among the prepared muffin cups and sprinkle with shredded cheese.

10. Bake in the preheated oven until the cheese is melted and the filling is bubbly, for about 15 to 20 minutes.

11. Top with diced avocado and garnish with chopped cilantro.

12. Serve with lime wedges and lime crema on the side.

Total Cook Time:45mins

CHAPTER 4

Healthy Snacks Recipes

Explore a variety of plant-based snacks designed to support prostate health while tantalizing your taste buds. Each delicious bite satisfies cravings and helps fortify your body against prostate cancer.

Broccoli Hummus

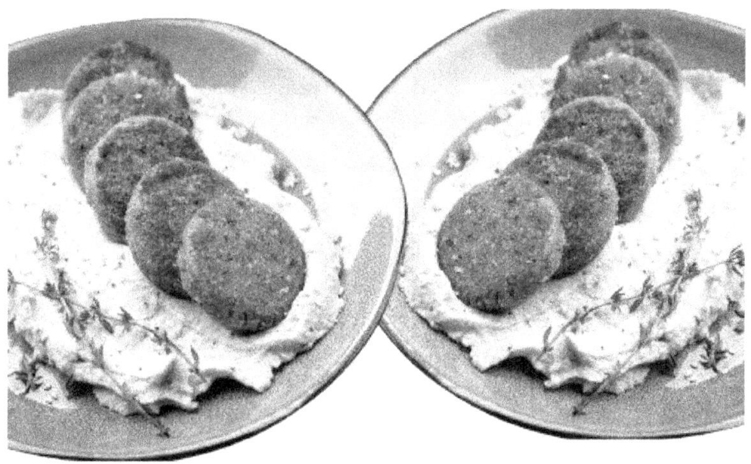

Ingredients

- 250g (9oz) broccoli florets (about 3 cups)
- 2 cloves of garlic, roughly chopped

- 1 unwaxed lemon (zest and juice)
- 75ml (3 fl oz) olive oil (5 tablespoons)
- 2 tablespoons of tahini (or almond/pistachio butter)
- 2 tablespoons of fresh parsley
- ½ teaspoon of salt
- ½ teaspoon of pepper
- 1 tablespoon of toasted sesame seeds (optional for garnish)

Instructions

1. Cut the broccoli into small florets.
2. Bring water to a boil in a pot and sprinkle in a pinch of salt.
3. Cook the broccoli in the boiling water for 5 minutes.
4. Use a slotted spoon or sieve to remove the broccoli from the water and place it in a food processor.
5. Add the broccoli to the food processor with the garlic, lemon zest, lemon juice, tahini (or nut butter), parsley, salt, and pepper.
6. Gradually pour in the olive oil while blending until smooth.
7. Move the mixture to a serving dish.

8. Sprinkle toasted sesame seeds on top (If using).

9. Drizzle with extra olive oil and garnish with additional parsley.

10. You can Serve it with Rye whole grain bread, oatcakes, or whole grain crackers

Total Time:15mins

Berry Smoothie

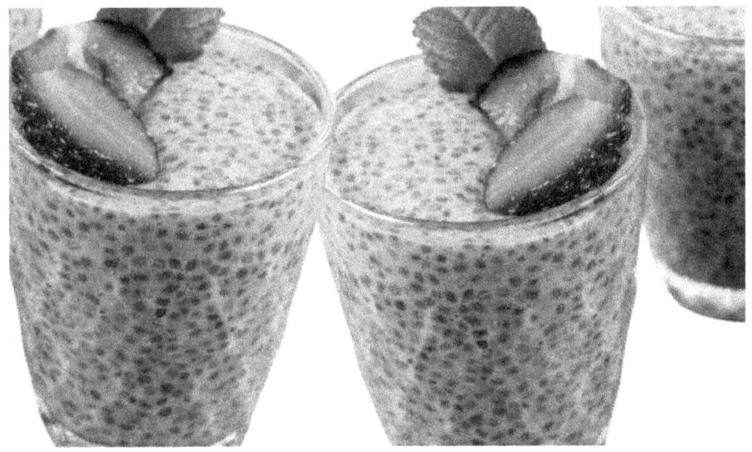

Ingredients:

- 1 cup of assorted berries (fresh or frozen)
- 1 banana
- 1 cup of almond milk
- 1 tablespoon of chia seeds

Instructions

1. Place the mixed berries, banana slices, almond milk, and chia seeds into a blender.
2. Blend all the ingredients quickly until the mixture is smooth and creamy. If the smoothie is too thick, incorporate additional almond milk.
3. Pour the smoothie into a glass.
4. Drink immediately for the best taste and freshness.

Total Time:5mins

Roasted Chickpeas

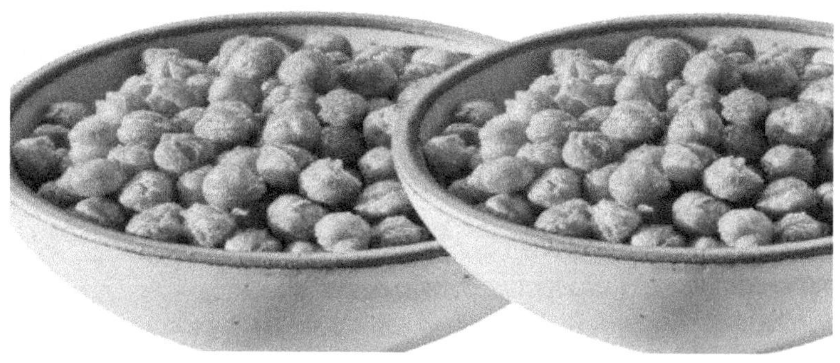

Ingredients:

*   1 (15 ounces) can of chickpeas, drained and rinsed
*   1 tablespoon of olive oil

- ¼ teaspoon of kosher salt (or adjusted to taste)
- ¼ teaspoon of smoked paprika
- ¼ teaspoon of black pepper
- ⅛ teaspoon of cayenne pepper (or to taste)
- ⅛ teaspoon of garlic powder

Instructions:

1. Preheat the oven to 450°F (220°C).
2. Drain and rinse the chickpeas.
3. Please place them in a bowl and blot with a paper towel to dry.
4. Toss the chickpeas with olive oil in the bowl.
5. Add salt, smoked paprika, black pepper, cayenne pepper, and garlic powder. Toss to coat evenly.
6. Spread the seasoned chickpeas on a rimmed baking sheet in a single layer.
7. Roast in the preheated oven for 30 to 40 minutes until browned and crunchy. Observe to avoid burning.
8. Cool and Enjoy: Let the chickpeas cool slightly before serving.

Prep Time:10 mins, Cook Time:20 mins, Additional Time:2 hrs, Total Time:2 hrs 30 mins

Kale Chips

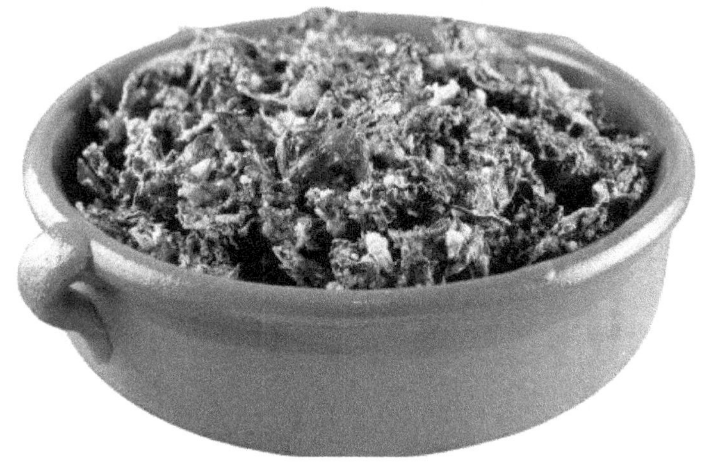

Ingredients:

- 1 bunch of kale
- 1 tablespoon of extra-virgin olive oil
- 1 tablespoon of sherry vinegar
- Sea salt, to taste

Instructions:

1. Preheat oven to 300°F (150°C).
2. Remove the inner ribs from the kale and tear the leaves into small pieces (like potato chips). Wash and dry thoroughly.

3. Place kale in a large resealable bag. Add half the olive oil, seal the bag, and massage to coat evenly. Add the remaining oil and massage again.
4. Add vinegar, reseal the bag, and shake well.
5. Spread kale on a baking sheet.
6. Bake for about 35 minutes, until mostly crisp.
7. Season with salt and serve immediately.

Total Time: 50 mins

Quinoa Salad

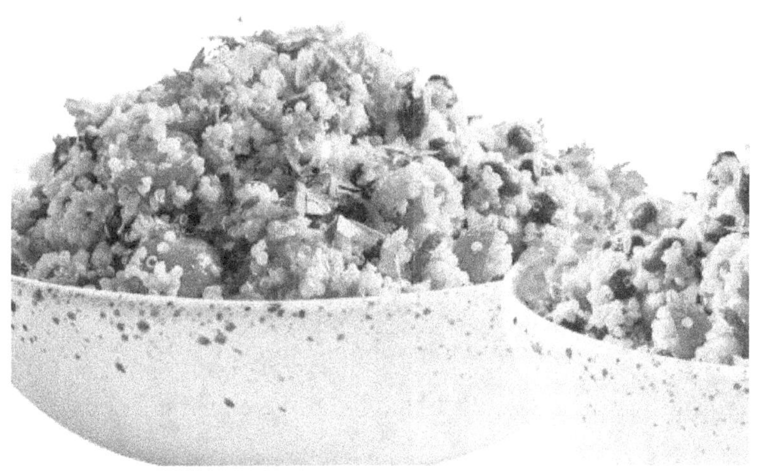

Ingredients

- 2 cups of water
- 1 cup of quinoa

- ¼ cup of extra-virgin olive oil

- Juice of 2 limes

- 2 teaspoons of ground cumin

- 1 teaspoon of salt

- ½ teaspoon of red pepper flakes, or adjust to your preference

- 1 ½ cups of halved cherry tomatoes

- 1 (15-ounce) can of black beans, drained and rinsed

- 5 green onions, finely chopped

- ¼ cup of chopped fresh cilantro

- Sea Salt and ground black pepper to taste

Instructions:

1. In a saucepan, bring the water and quinoa to a boil. Reduce heat to medium-low, cover, and simmer for 10 to 15 minutes until the quinoa is tender and the water is absorbed. Set aside to cool.

2. As the quinoa cools, blend the olive oil, lime juice, cumin, salt, and red pepper flakes in a small bowl.

3. Combine the cooled quinoa, cherry tomatoes, black beans, and green onions in a large bowl.

4. Drizzle the dressing over the mixture and toss gently to ensure an even coating. Add the cilantro and season with salt and black pepper according to your taste preferences.

5. Serve immediately or chill in the refrigerator before serving.

Total Time:35 mins

Almond Butter Banana Toast

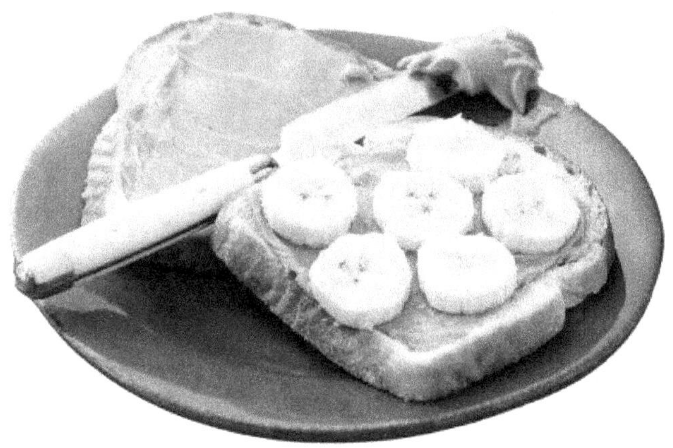

Ingredients:

- 1 slice of whole-grain bread
- 1 tablespoon of almond butter
- 1 banana

Instructions:

1. Toast the bread until it reaches your desired level of crispness.
2. Spread a generous layer of almond butter on the warm toast.
3. Slice the banana and arrange the slices evenly on top.

Total Time: 5 minutes

Black Bean Avocado Salsa

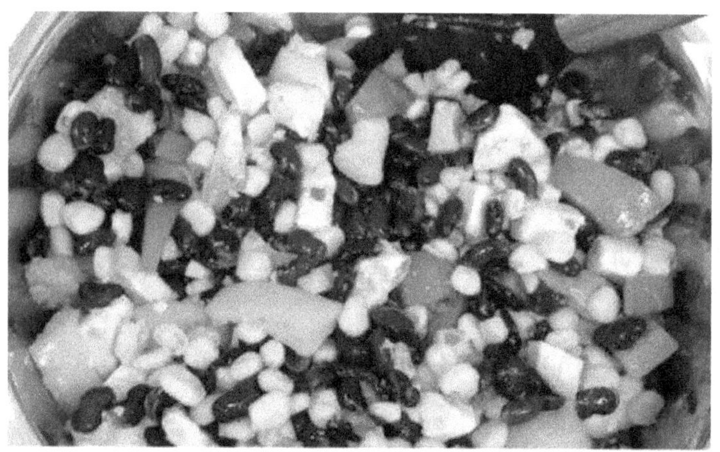

Ingredients:

- One can of black beans (15 ounces), rinsed and drained

- can whole kernel sweet corn (11 ounces), drained

- 4 Roma (plum) tomatoes, seeded and chopped

- 1 small red bell pepper, diced
- 1 jalapeno pepper, seeded and minced
- ⅓ cup of fresh cilantro, chopped
- ¼ cup of red onion, diced
- ¼ cup of fresh lime juice
- tablespoons of red wine vinegar
- 1 teaspoon of salt
- ½ teaspoon of ground black pepper
- avocados, diced

Instructions:

1. Combine the black beans, corn, tomatoes, red bell pepper, jalapeno pepper, cilantro, and red onion in a large bowl.
2. Add the lime juice, red wine vinegar, salt, and black pepper to the mixture and stir well.
3. Gently fold in the diced avocados.
4. Cover the bowl with plastic wrap, ensuring it is in direct contact with the salsa.
5. Refrigerate for a minimum of 2 hours before serving to chill.

Prep Time:15 mins, Additional Time:2 hrs

Total Time:2 hrs 15 mins

Chapter 5

Sweet Treats - Dessert Recipes

Discover delicious anti-prostate cancer dessert recipes that blend flavor and health, featuring ingredients known for their cancer-fighting properties. Treat yourself to the deliciousness that nurtures your well-being.

Berry Chia Pudding

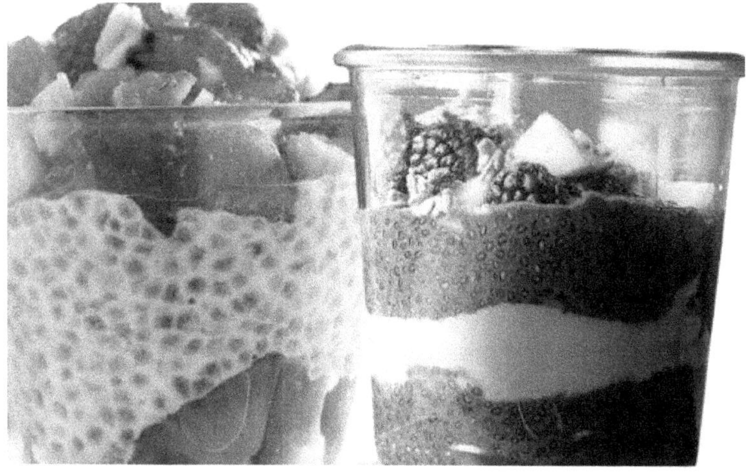

Ingredients:

- 1 ¾ cups of mixed blackberries, raspberries, and diced mango (fresh or frozen) divided

- one cup of unsweetened almond milk or any plant-based milk of your choice
- ¼ cup of chia seeds
- 1 tablespoon of pure maple syrup
- ¾ teaspoon of vanilla extract
- ½ cup of whole-milk plain Greek yogurt
- ¼ cup of granola

Instructions:

1. Blend 1 ¼ cups of the fruit and milk until smooth. Pour into a medium bowl and mix in the chia seeds, maple syrup, and vanilla. Cover and refrigerate for at least 8 hours or up to 3 days.
2. Divide the pudding into 2 bowls. Layer each serving with ¼ cup of the remaining fruit, ¼ cup of yogurt, and 2 tablespoons of granola.
   Prep Time:5 mins, Additional Time:8 hrs Total Time:8 hrs 5 mins

Dark Chocolate Avocado Mousse

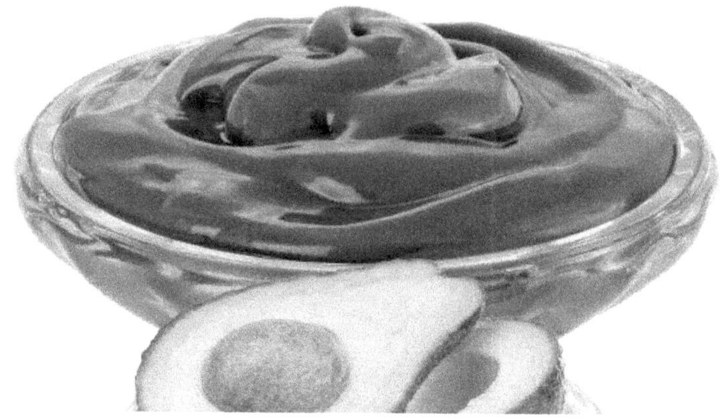

Ingredients:

- The flesh of 2 ripe avocados (240g)
- 1/4 cup of regular cocoa powder
- 1/4 cup of Dutch cocoa powder
- 3-4 tablespoons of almond milk
- 1/2 teaspoon of pure vanilla extract
- 1/8 teaspoon of salt
- Sweetener of choice to taste (e.g., 1/4 cup pure maple syrup)

Instructions

1. Scoop the flesh from 2 ripe avocados.

2. Add the avocado, regular cocoa powder, Dutch cocoa powder, almond milk, vanilla extract, salt, and sweetener to a blender or food processor.

3. Blend until completely smooth and creamy.

4. Chill in the refrigerator before serving for a thicker texture.

Total Time: 5 mins

Banana Ice Cream

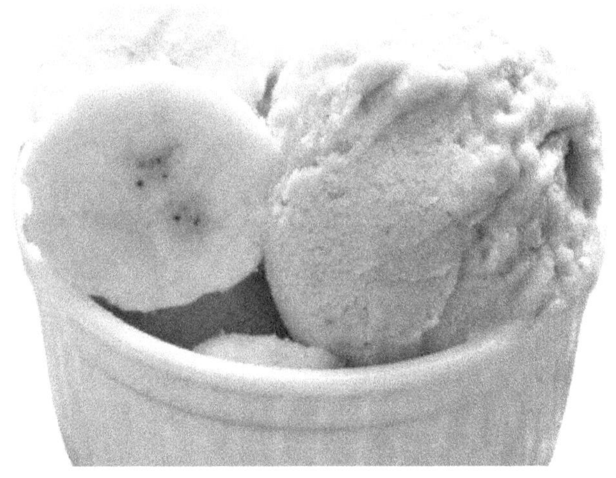

Ingredients

- 2 ripe bananas
- 1/4 cup of almond milk

Instructions

1. Peel and slice the bananas. Please place them in the freezer until fully frozen.
2. In a blender, combine the frozen banana slices and almond milk. Blend until smooth and creamy.
3. Enjoy immediately as a soft-serve treat, or freeze for an additional hour for a firmer texture.

Total Time: 5 mins

Apple Cinnamon Oatmeal

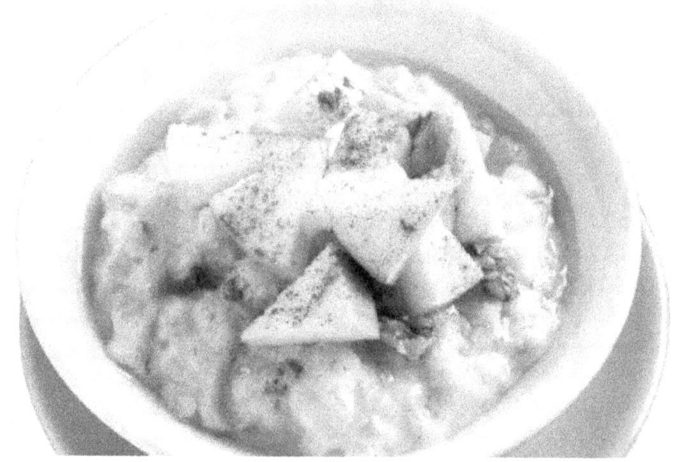

Ingredients

- 1 cup of water

- 1/4 cup of apple juice

- 1 apple, cored and chopped

- 2/3 cup of rolled oats

- 1 teaspoon of ground cinnamon

- 1 cup of plant-based milk (like almond milk)

Instructions

1. Mix the water, apple juice, and chopped apple in a saucepan.
2. Heat the mixture over high heat until it boils.
3. Stir in the rolled oats and ground cinnamon.
4. Return the mixture to a boil, then reduce the heat to low. Let it simmer until thickened, about 3 minutes.
5. Spoon the oatmeal into serving bowls and add the plant-based milk. Enjoy warm. You can add fresh apples if you like.

Total Time:10 mins

Pumpkin Spice Smoothie

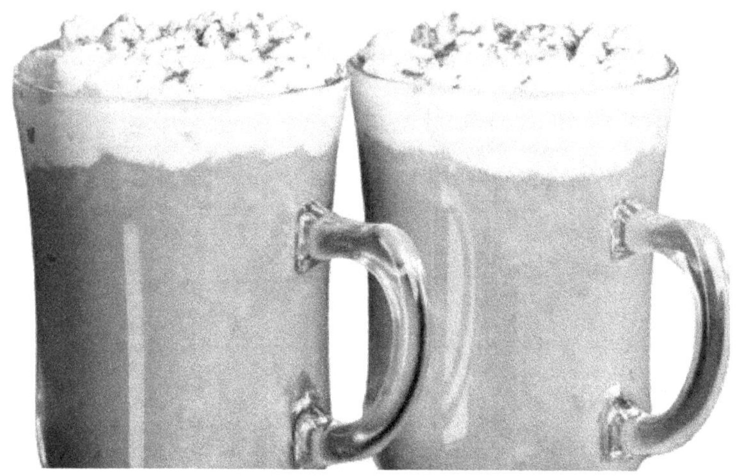

Ingredients

- 1 frozen banana
- 1/2 cup of plain or vanilla yogurt
- 1/2 cup of pumpkin puree
- 1/2 cup of unsweetened almond milk
- 1 tablespoon of almond or pecan butter
- 1 teaspoon of vanilla extract
- 1/2 teaspoon of ground cinnamon
- Pinch of nutmeg
- Pinch of ginger
- Pinch of allspice

Instructions

1. Combine Ingredients: Add the frozen banana, yogurt, pumpkin puree, almond milk, almond or pecan butter, vanilla extract, ground cinnamon, nutmeg, ginger, and allspice into a blender.
2. Blend: Blend everything until smooth.
3. Serve: Pour into a glass and enjoy.

Total Time: 10minutes

Coconut Date Balls

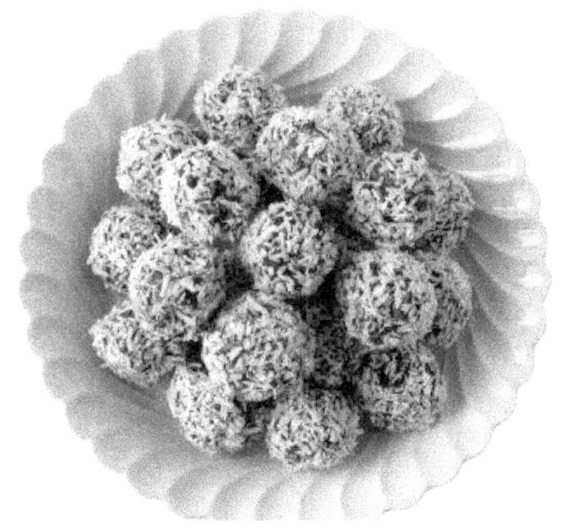

Ingredients

* 10-12 Medjool dates

- 2 cups of pecans

- Pinch of sea salt

- 1/4 cup of desiccated coconut

Instructions

1. Pit the Medjool dates and soak them in warm water for 10 minutes until they soften.
2. Place the pitted dates and pecans in a large food processor. Blend on high until a thick, sticky dough forms.
3. Scoop about 1-2 tablespoons of the mixture and roll it into a ball using your hands.
4. If desired, let the balls set in the fridge for 5 minutes. Then, roll them in desiccated coconut, pressing gently to ensure they stick.
5. Enjoy immediately or store in the fridge. You can make about 12-14 bites.

Total Time: 10minutes

Practical tips and advice to improve your prostate health

Eat a Plant-Based Diet: Focus on vegetables, fruits, whole grains, and legumes to boost your intake of antioxidants and fiber, which support prostate health.

Incorporate Healthy Fats: Opt for sources of healthy fats like olive oil, avocados, nuts, and seeds instead of saturated fats.

Stay Hydrated: Drink plenty of water throughout the day to maintain overall health and aid in detoxification.

Exercise Regularly: Engage in at least 30 minutes of physical activity most days of the week to improve circulation and reduce inflammation.

Limit Red Meat and Dairy: Reduce consumption of red meat and dairy products, which have been linked to prostate health issues.

Include Cruciferous Vegetables: Add broccoli, cauliflower, kale, and Brussels sprouts to your diet, as they contain compounds that support prostate health.

Avoid Smoking and Excessive Alcohol: These habits can increase the risk of prostate problems and other health issues.

Manage Stress: Practice stress-reducing techniques such as meditation, yoga, or deep breathing exercises to maintain hormonal balance.

Regular Screenings: Schedule regular check-ups with your healthcare provider to monitor prostate health and catch any issues early.

Maintain a Healthy Weight: Achieve and maintain a healthy weight through a balanced diet and regular exercise to reduce the risk of prostate disease.

Stay Positive: Maintain a positive outlook on life, as a positive mindset can improve overall well-being and aid in recovery and health maintenance.

CONCLUSION

Starting a plant-based diet isn't just about food; it's a big step towards a healthier and happier life. With the recipes in this cookbook, you hold the key to creating delicious and nourishing meals that support prostate health and reduce cancer risks.

Every meal becomes a powerful opportunity to cherish your body and fight disease. By choosing plant-based foods, you're making a positive change for your health and taking charge of your well-being.

Don't forget that exercising regularly and seeing your doctor for check-ups are super important, too! Moving your body keeps you strong and happy, and going for check-ups helps catch any problems early. It's like giving yourself a big hug of self-care and ensuring you're staying your best self!

Thank you for letting this book be part of your journey. Here's to a vibrant, healthy life filled with fresh, wholesome meals!

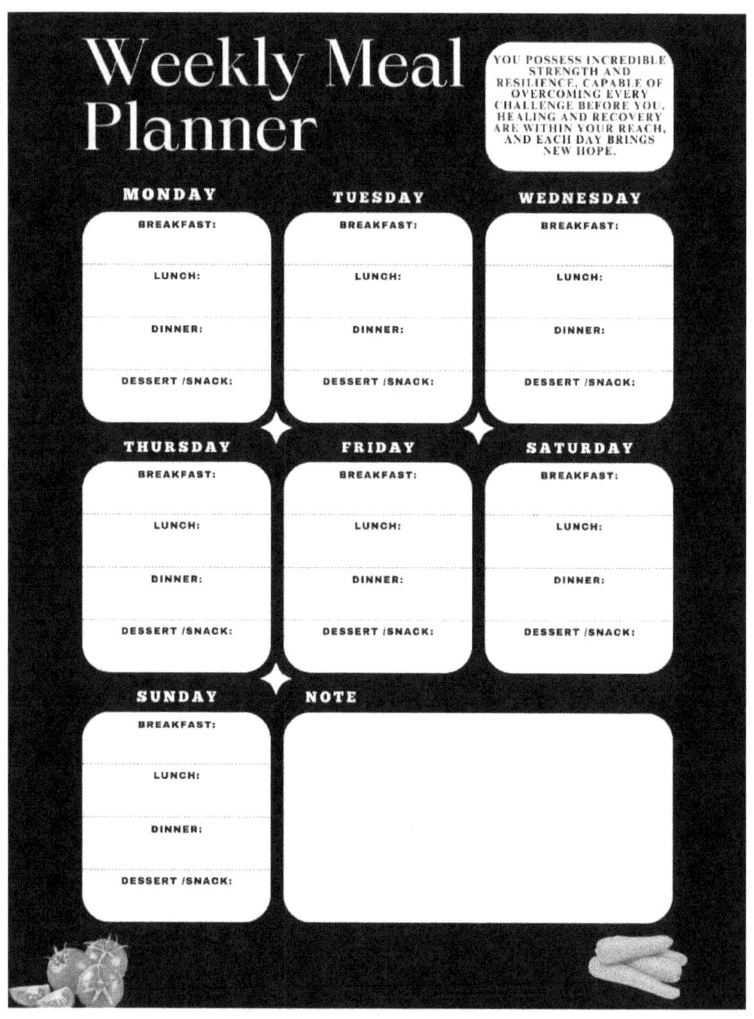

Weekly Meal Planner

YOU POSSESS INCREDIBLE STRENGTH AND RESILIENCE, CAPABLE OF OVERCOMING EVERY CHALLENGE BEFORE YOU. HEALING AND RECOVERY ARE WITHIN YOUR REACH, AND EACH DAY BRINGS NEW HOPE.

MONDAY
BREAKFAST:
LUNCH:
DINNER:
DESSERT /SNACK:

TUESDAY
BREAKFAST:
LUNCH:
DINNER:
DESSERT /SNACK:

WEDNESDAY
BREAKFAST:
LUNCH:
DINNER:
DESSERT /SNACK:

THURSDAY
BREAKFAST:
LUNCH:
DINNER:
DESSERT /SNACK:

FRIDAY
BREAKFAST:
LUNCH:
DINNER:
DESSERT /SNACK:

SATURDAY
BREAKFAST:
LUNCH:
DINNER:
DESSERT /SNACK:

SUNDAY
BREAKFAST:
LUNCH:
DINNER:
DESSERT /SNACK:

NOTE

Weekly Meal Planner

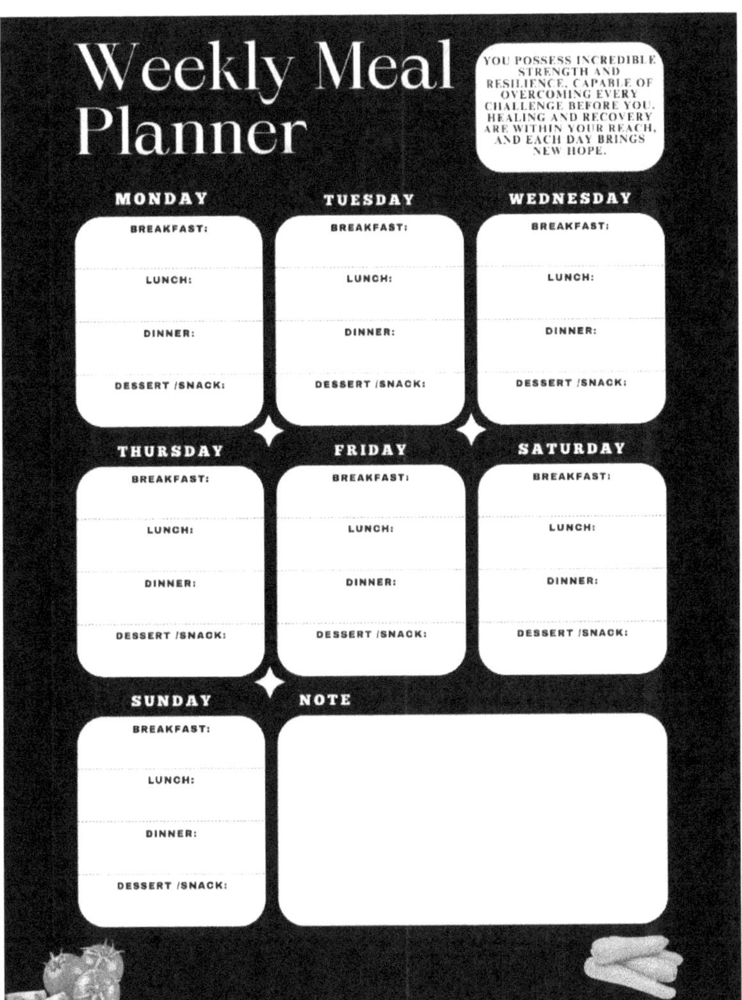

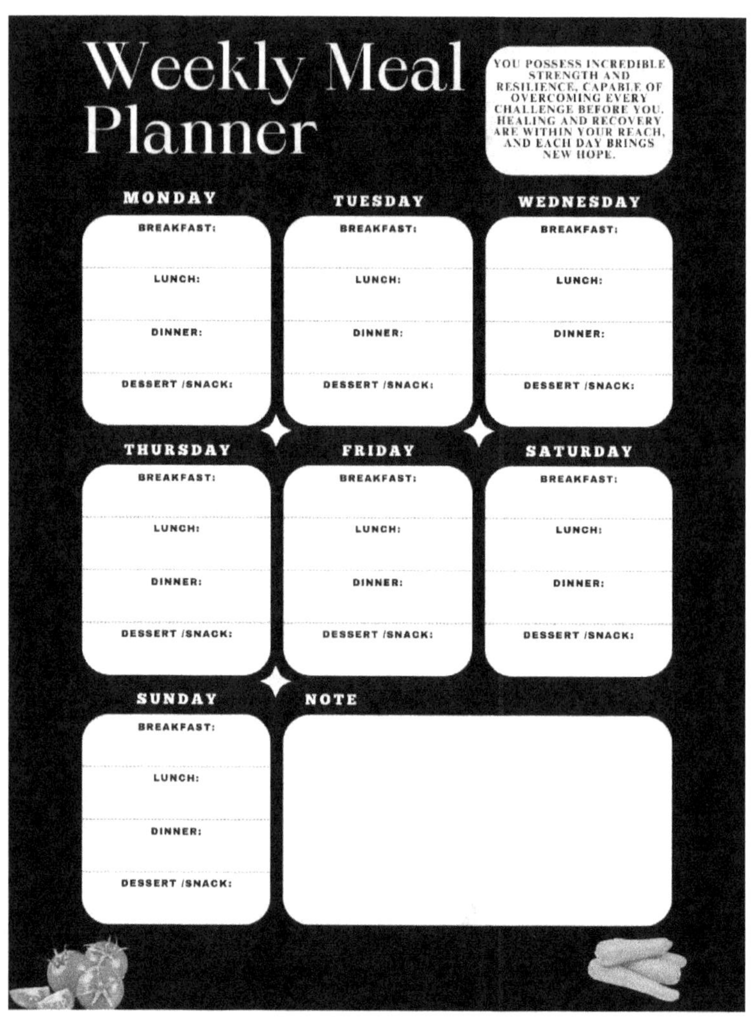

Weekly Meal Planner

YOU POSSESS INCREDIBLE STRENGTH AND RESILIENCE, CAPABLE OF OVERCOMING EVERY CHALLENGE BEFORE YOU. HEALING AND RECOVERY ARE WITHIN YOUR REACH, AND EACH DAY BRINGS NEW HOPE.

MONDAY
BREAKFAST:
LUNCH:
DINNER:
DESSERT /SNACK:

TUESDAY
BREAKFAST:
LUNCH:
DINNER:
DESSERT /SNACK:

WEDNESDAY
BREAKFAST:
LUNCH:
DINNER:
DESSERT /SNACK:

THURSDAY
BREAKFAST:
LUNCH:
DINNER:
DESSERT /SNACK:

FRIDAY
BREAKFAST:
LUNCH:
DINNER:
DESSERT /SNACK:

SATURDAY
BREAKFAST:
LUNCH:
DINNER:
DESSERT /SNACK:

SUNDAY
BREAKFAST:
LUNCH:
DINNER:
DESSERT /SNACK:

NOTE

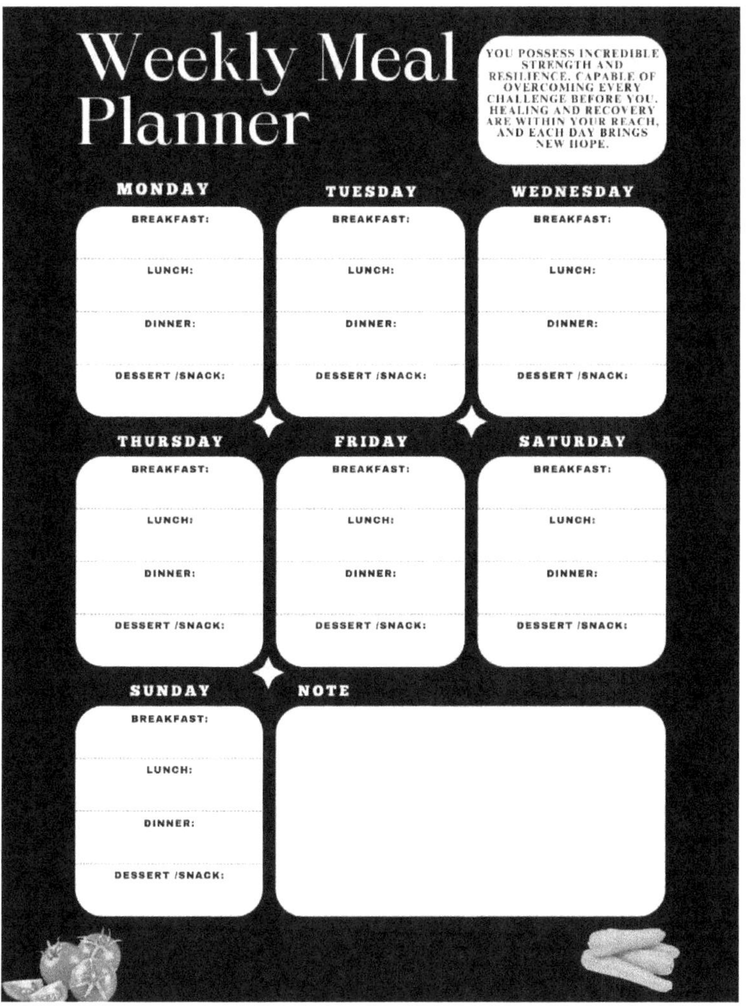

Weekly Meal Planner

MONDAY

BREAKFAST:

LUNCH:

DINNER:

DESSERT /SNACK:

TUESDAY

BREAKFAST:

LUNCH:

DINNER:

DESSERT /SNACK:

WEDNESDAY

BREAKFAST:

LUNCH:

DINNER:

DESSERT /SNACK:

THURSDAY

BREAKFAST:

LUNCH:

DINNER:

DESSERT /SNACK:

FRIDAY

BREAKFAST:

LUNCH:

DINNER:

DESSERT /SNACK:

SATURDAY

BREAKFAST:

LUNCH:

DINNER:

DESSERT /SNACK:

SUNDAY

BREAKFAST:

LUNCH:

DINNER:

DESSERT /SNACK:

NOTE

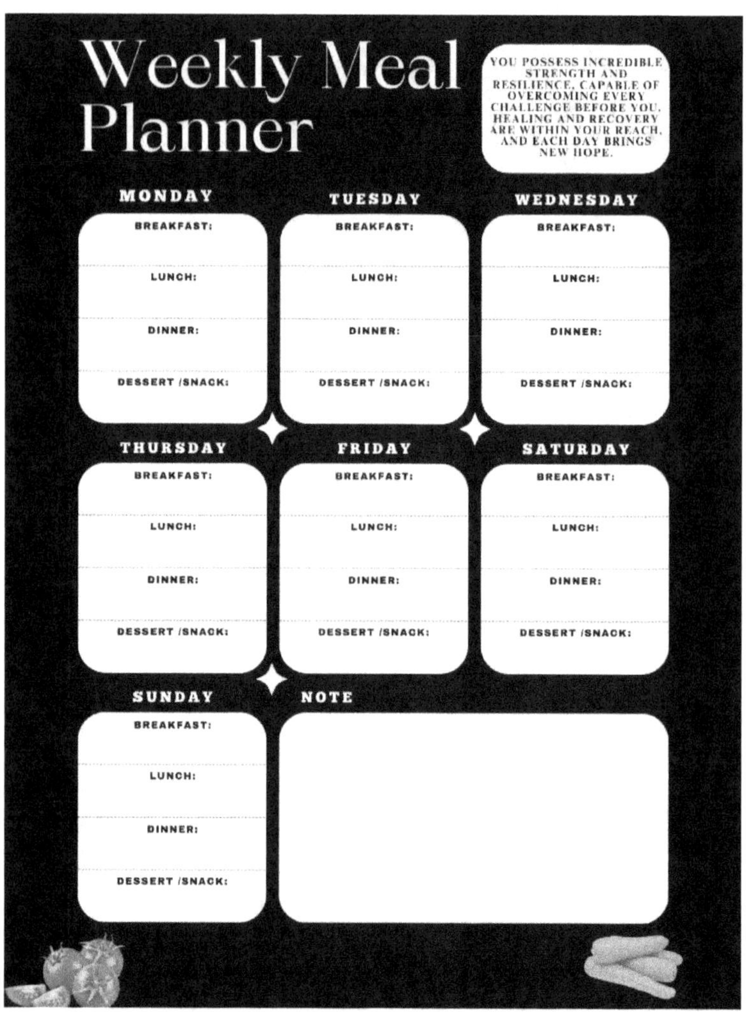

Weekly Meal Planner

YOU POSSESS INCREDIBLE STRENGTH AND RESILIENCE, CAPABLE OF OVERCOMING EVERY CHALLENGE BEFORE YOU. HEALING AND RECOVERY ARE WITHIN YOUR REACH, AND EACH DAY BRINGS NEW HOPE.

MONDAY
BREAKFAST:
LUNCH:
DINNER:
DESSERT /SNACK:

TUESDAY
BREAKFAST:
LUNCH:
DINNER:
DESSERT /SNACK:

WEDNESDAY
BREAKFAST:
LUNCH:
DINNER:
DESSERT /SNACK:

THURSDAY
BREAKFAST:
LUNCH:
DINNER:
DESSERT /SNACK:

FRIDAY
BREAKFAST:
LUNCH:
DINNER:
DESSERT /SNACK:

SATURDAY
BREAKFAST:
LUNCH:
DINNER:
DESSERT /SNACK:

SUNDAY
BREAKFAST:
LUNCH:
DINNER:
DESSERT /SNACK:

NOTE

Weekly Meal Planner

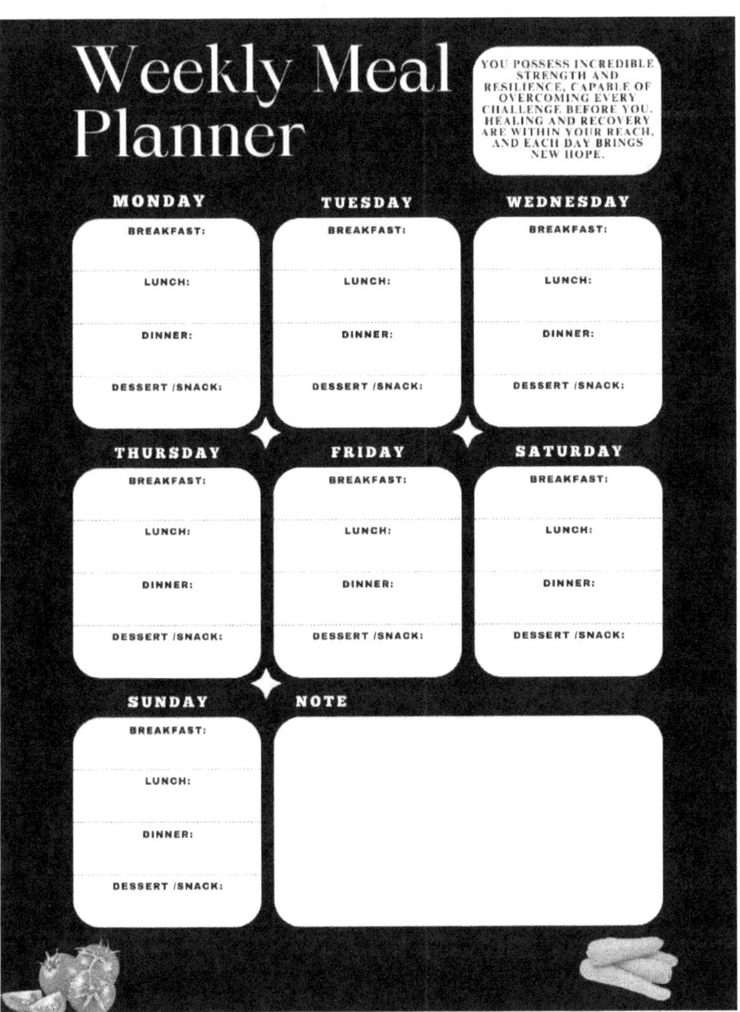

Weekly Meal Planner

YOU POSSESS INCREDIBLE STRENGTH AND RESILIENCE, CAPABLE OF OVERCOMING EVERY CHALLENGE BEFORE YOU. HEALING AND RECOVERY ARE WITHIN YOUR REACH, AND EACH DAY BRINGS NEW HOPE.

MONDAY

BREAKFAST:

LUNCH:

DINNER:

DESSERT /SNACK:

TUESDAY

BREAKFAST:

LUNCH:

DINNER:

DESSERT /SNACK:

WEDNESDAY

BREAKFAST:

LUNCH:

DINNER:

DESSERT /SNACK:

THURSDAY

BREAKFAST:

LUNCH:

DINNER:

DESSERT /SNACK:

FRIDAY

BREAKFAST:

LUNCH:

DINNER:

DESSERT /SNACK:

SATURDAY

BREAKFAST:

LUNCH:

DINNER:

DESSERT /SNACK:

SUNDAY

BREAKFAST:

LUNCH:

DINNER:

DESSERT /SNACK:

NOTE

Weekly Meal Planner

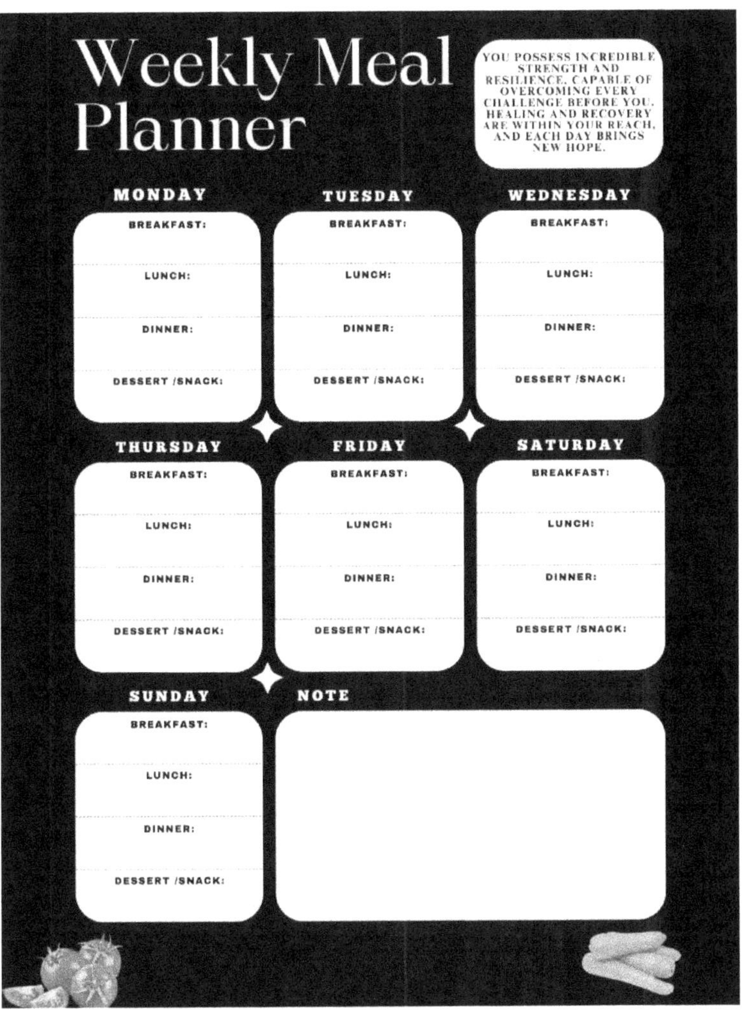

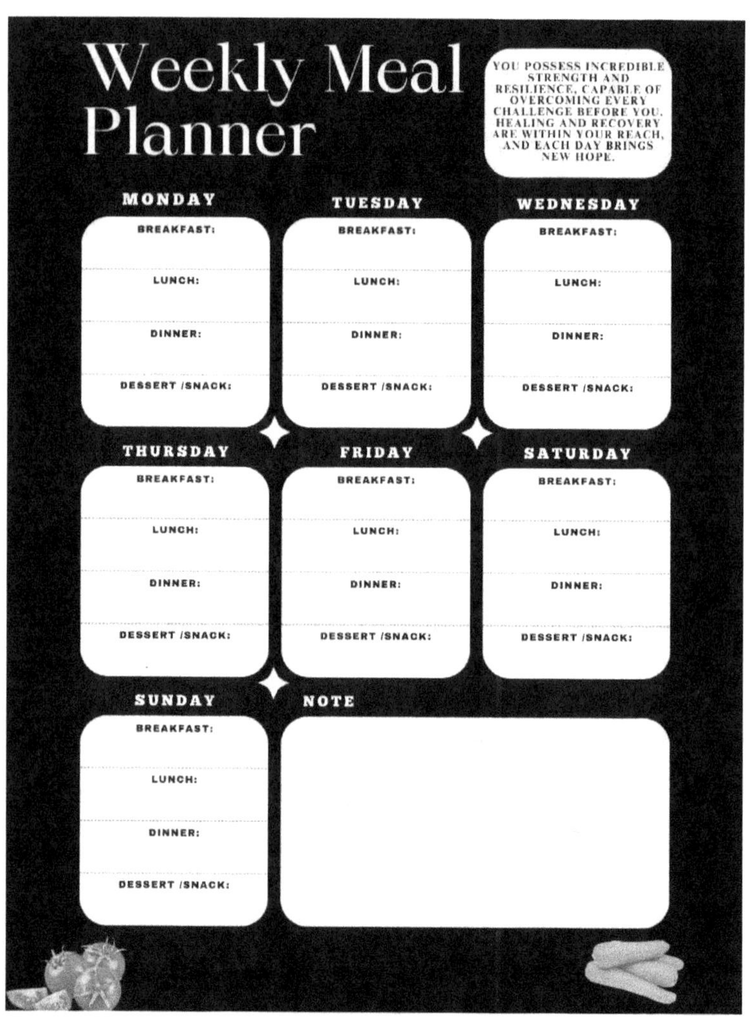

Weekly Meal Planner

YOU POSSESS INCREDIBLE
STRENGTH AND
RESILIENCE, CAPABLE OF
OVERCOMING EVERY
CHALLENGE BEFORE YOU.
HEALING AND RECOVERY
ARE WITHIN YOUR REACH,
AND EACH DAY BRINGS
NEW HOPE.

MONDAY
BREAKFAST:
LUNCH:
DINNER:
DESSERT /SNACK:

TUESDAY
BREAKFAST:
LUNCH:
DINNER:
DESSERT /SNACK:

WEDNESDAY
BREAKFAST:
LUNCH:
DINNER:
DESSERT /SNACK:

THURSDAY
BREAKFAST:
LUNCH:
DINNER:
DESSERT /SNACK:

FRIDAY
BREAKFAST:
LUNCH:
DINNER:
DESSERT /SNACK:

SATURDAY
BREAKFAST:
LUNCH:
DINNER:
DESSERT /SNACK:

SUNDAY
BREAKFAST:
LUNCH:
DINNER:
DESSERT /SNACK:

NOTE

Weekly Meal Planner

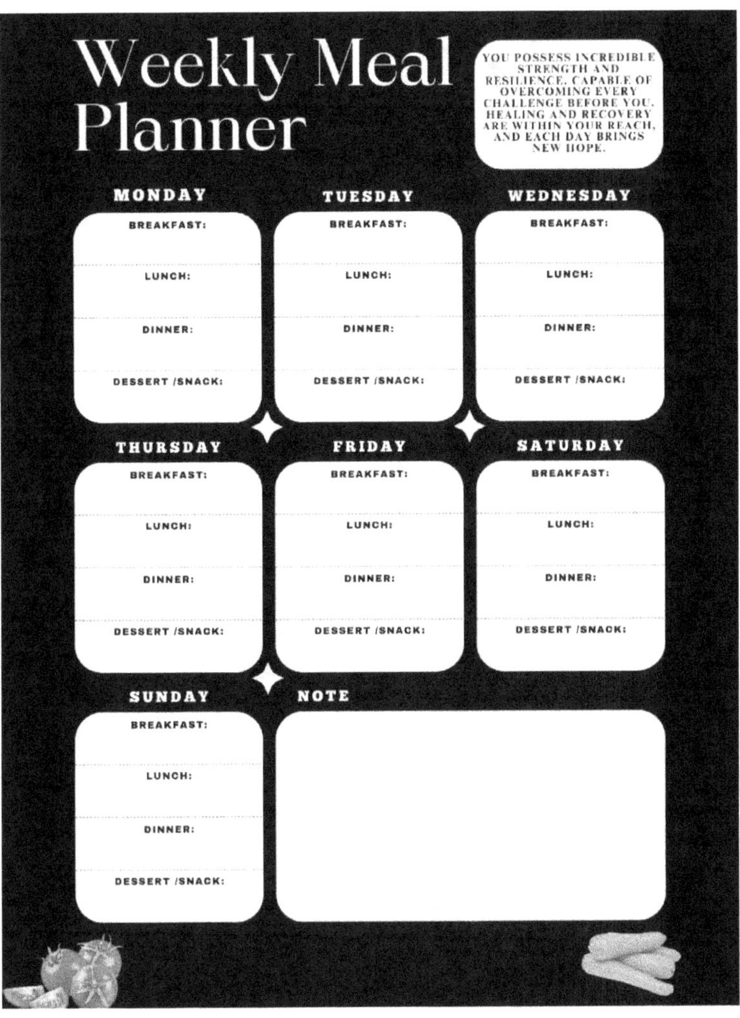

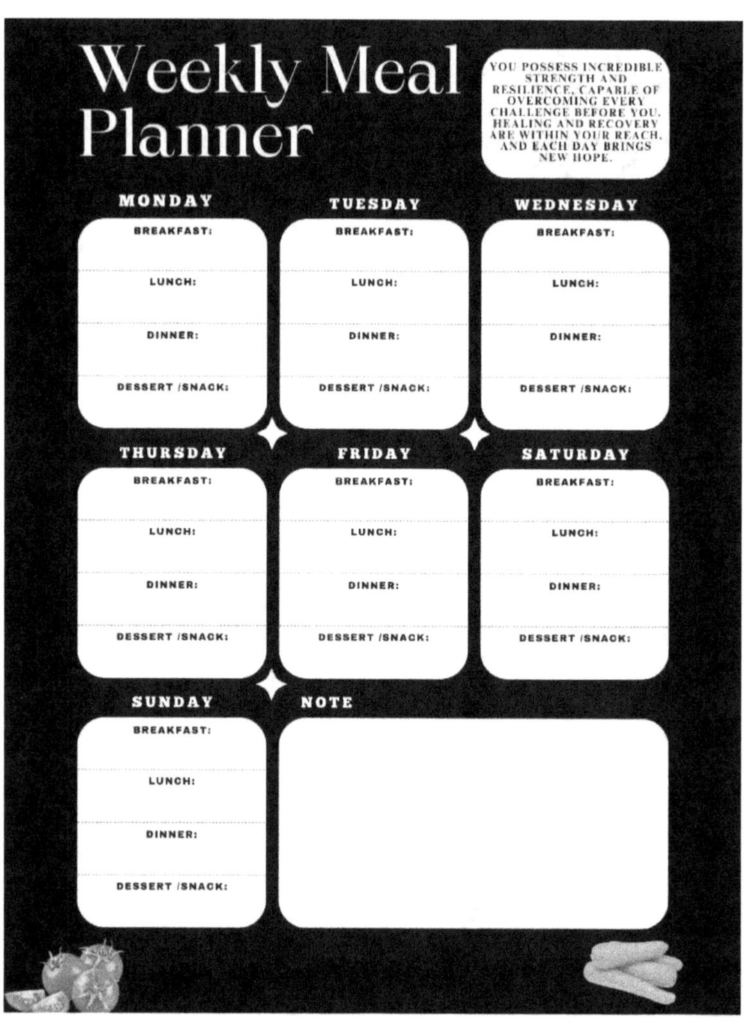

Weekly Meal Planner

MONDAY

BREAKFAST:

LUNCH:

DINNER:

DESSERT /SNACK:

TUESDAY

BREAKFAST:

LUNCH:

DINNER:

DESSERT /SNACK:

WEDNESDAY

BREAKFAST:

LUNCH:

DINNER:

DESSERT /SNACK:

THURSDAY

BREAKFAST:

LUNCH:

DINNER:

DESSERT /SNACK:

FRIDAY

BREAKFAST:

LUNCH:

DINNER:

DESSERT /SNACK:

SATURDAY

BREAKFAST:

LUNCH:

DINNER:

DESSERT /SNACK:

SUNDAY

BREAKFAST:

LUNCH:

DINNER:

DESSERT /SNACK:

NOTE

Weekly Meal Planner

YOU POSSESS INCREDIBLE STRENGTH AND RESILIENCE, CAPABLE OF OVERCOMING EVERY CHALLENGE BEFORE YOU. HEALING AND RECOVERY ARE WITHIN YOUR REACH, AND EACH DAY BRINGS NEW HOPE.

MONDAY

BREAKFAST:

LUNCH:

DINNER:

DESSERT /SNACK:

TUESDAY

BREAKFAST:

LUNCH:

DINNER:

DESSERT /SNACK:

WEDNESDAY

BREAKFAST:

LUNCH:

DINNER:

DESSERT /SNACK:

THURSDAY

BREAKFAST:

LUNCH:

DINNER:

DESSERT /SNACK:

FRIDAY

BREAKFAST:

LUNCH:

DINNER:

DESSERT /SNACK:

SATURDAY

BREAKFAST:

LUNCH:

DINNER:

DESSERT /SNACK:

SUNDAY

BREAKFAST:

LUNCH:

DINNER:

DESSERT /SNACK:

NOTE

Weekly Meal Planner

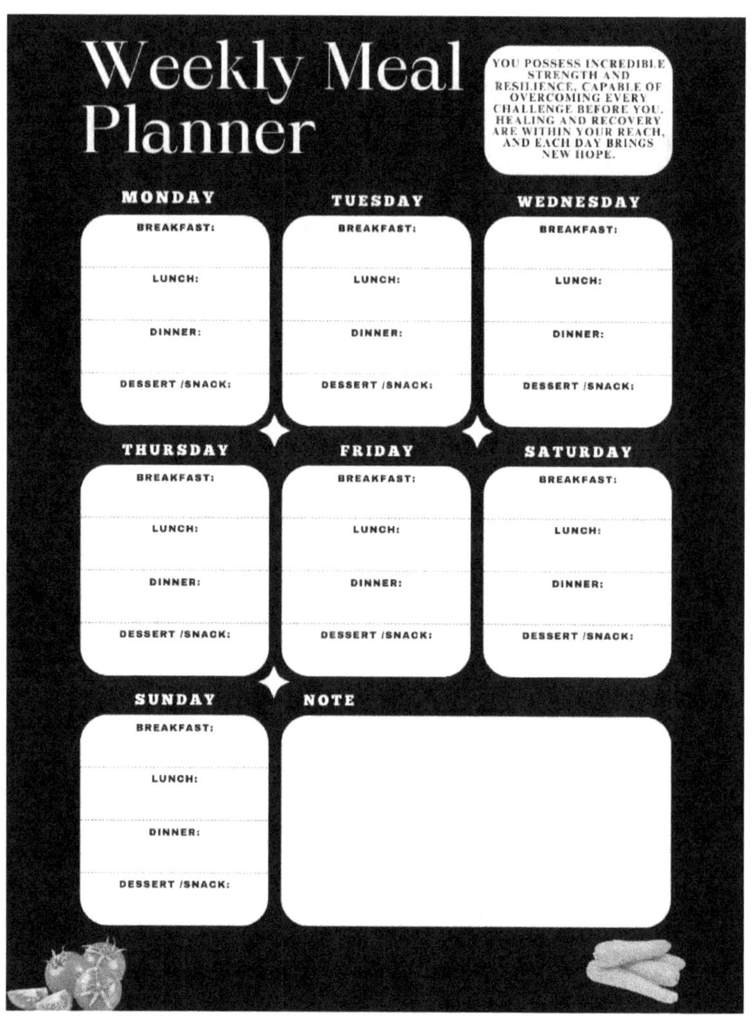

Weekly Meal Planner

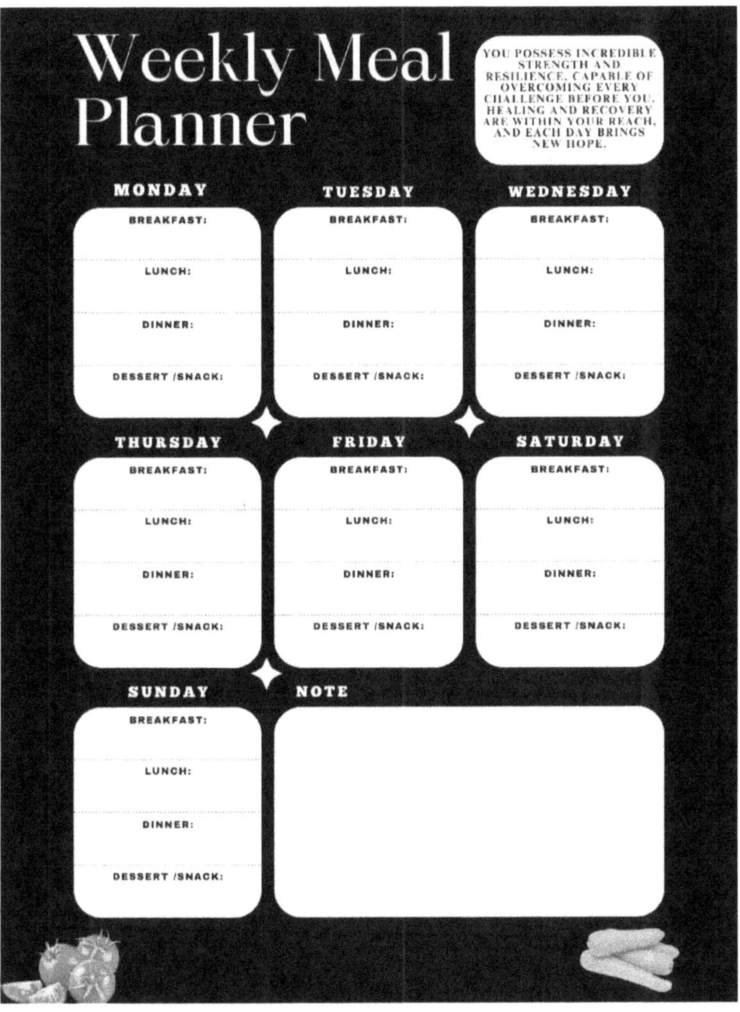

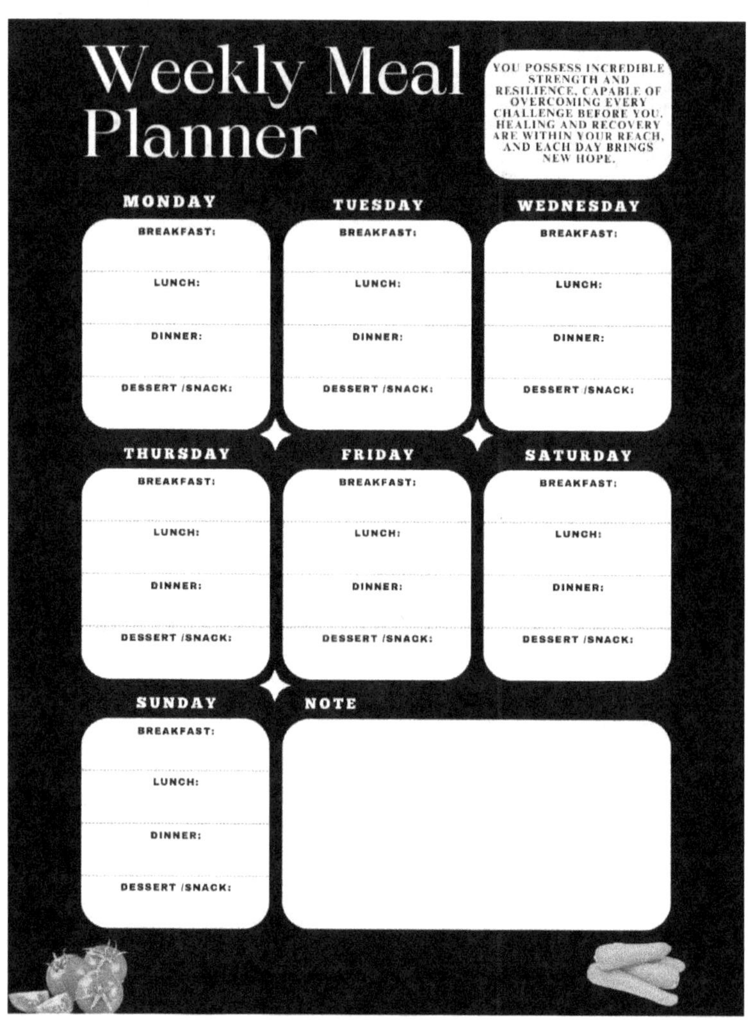

Weekly Meal Planner
YOU POSSESS INCREDIBLE STRENGTH AND RESILIENCE, CAPABLE OF OVERCOMING EVERY CHALLENGE BEFORE YOU. HEALING AND RECOVERY ARE WITHIN YOUR REACH, AND EACH DAY BRINGS NEW HOPE.
MONDAY
BREAKFAST:
LUNCH:
DINNER:
DESSERT /SNACK:
TUESDAY
BREAKFAST:
LUNCH:
DINNER:
DESSERT /SNACK:
WEDNESDAY
BREAKFAST:
LUNCH:
DINNER:
DESSERT /SNACK:
THURSDAY
BREAKFAST:
LUNCH:
DINNER:
DESSERT /SNACK:
FRIDAY
BREAKFAST:
LUNCH:
DINNER:
DESSERT /SNACK:
SATURDAY
BREAKFAST:
LUNCH:
DINNER:
DESSERT /SNACK:
SUNDAY
BREAKFAST:
LUNCH:
DINNER:
DESSERT /SNACK:
NOTE

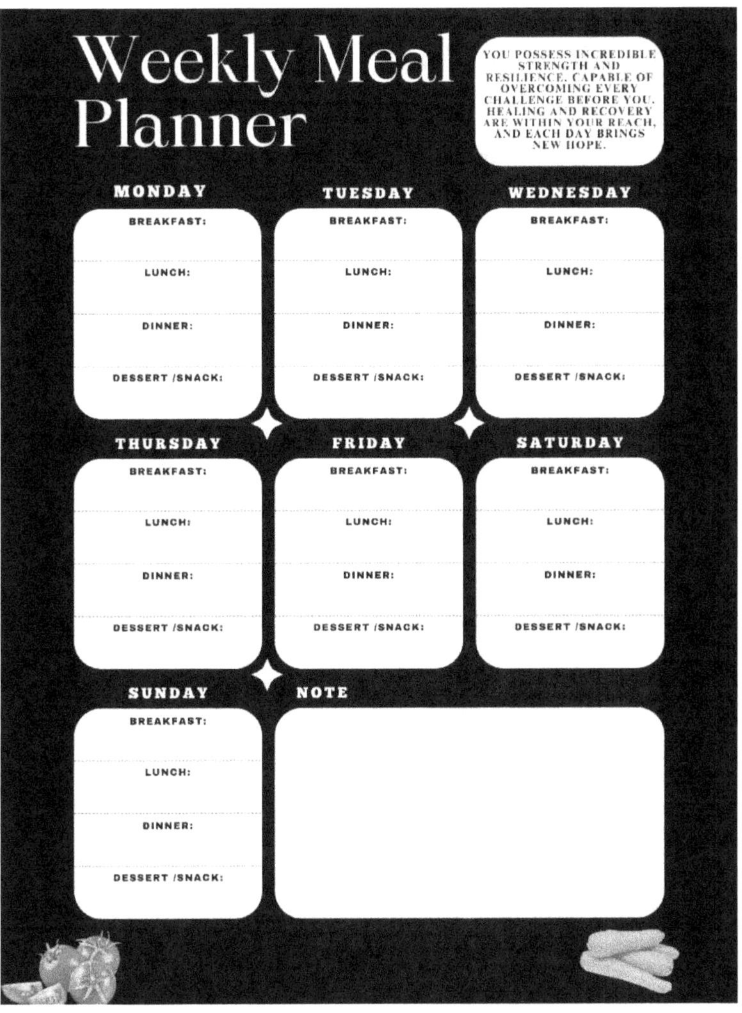

Weekly Meal Planner

YOU POSSESS INCREDIBLE STRENGTH AND RESILIENCE, CAPABLE OF OVERCOMING EVERY CHALLENGE BEFORE YOU. HEALING AND RECOVERY ARE WITHIN YOUR REACH, AND EACH DAY BRINGS NEW HOPE.

MONDAY
BREAKFAST:
LUNCH:
DINNER:
DESSERT /SNACK:

TUESDAY
BREAKFAST:
LUNCH:
DINNER:
DESSERT /SNACK:

WEDNESDAY
BREAKFAST:
LUNCH:
DINNER:
DESSERT /SNACK:

THURSDAY
BREAKFAST:
LUNCH:
DINNER:
DESSERT /SNACK:

FRIDAY
BREAKFAST:
LUNCH:
DINNER:
DESSERT /SNACK:

SATURDAY
BREAKFAST:
LUNCH:
DINNER:
DESSERT /SNACK:

SUNDAY
BREAKFAST:
LUNCH:
DINNER:
DESSERT /SNACK:

NOTE

Weekly Meal Planner

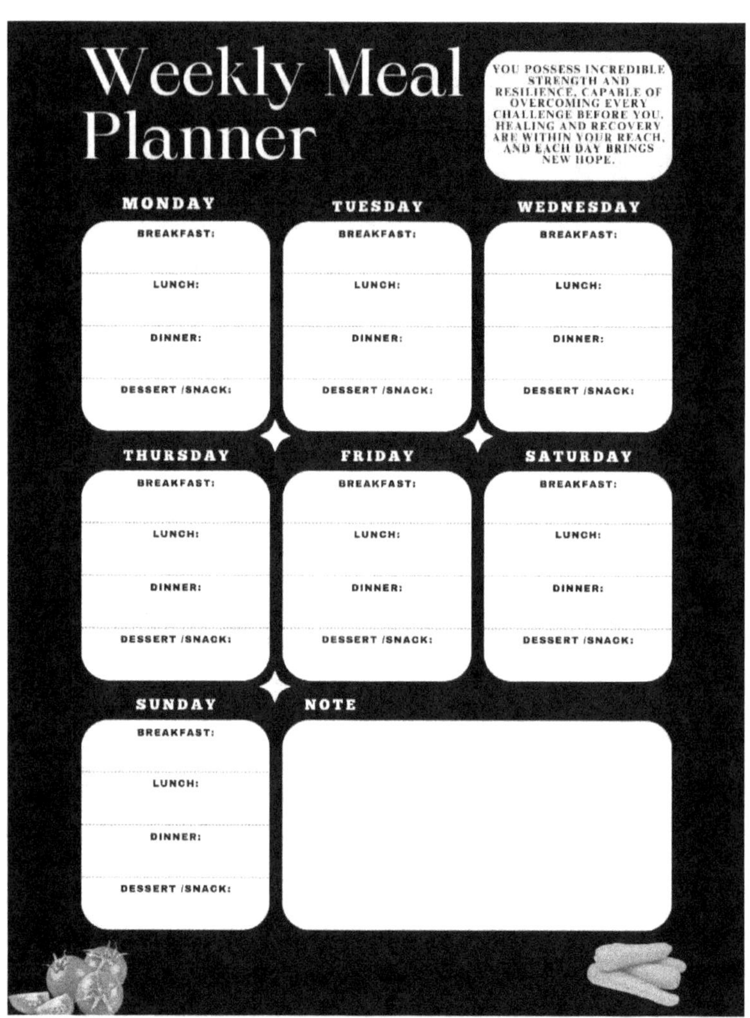

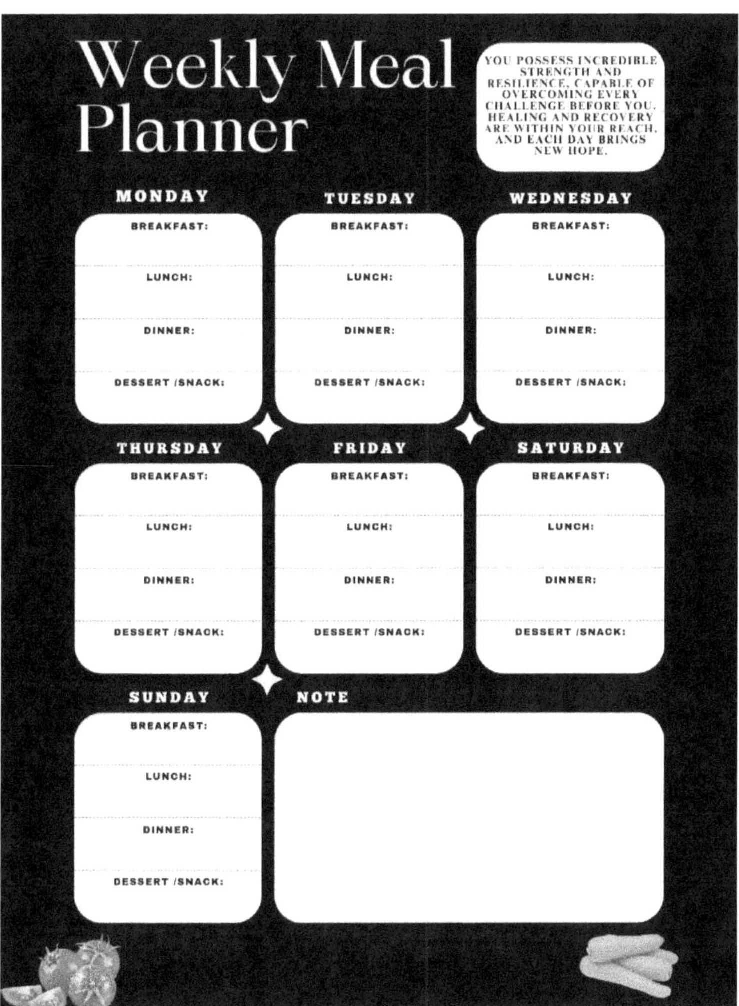

Weekly Meal Planner

Weekly Meal Planner

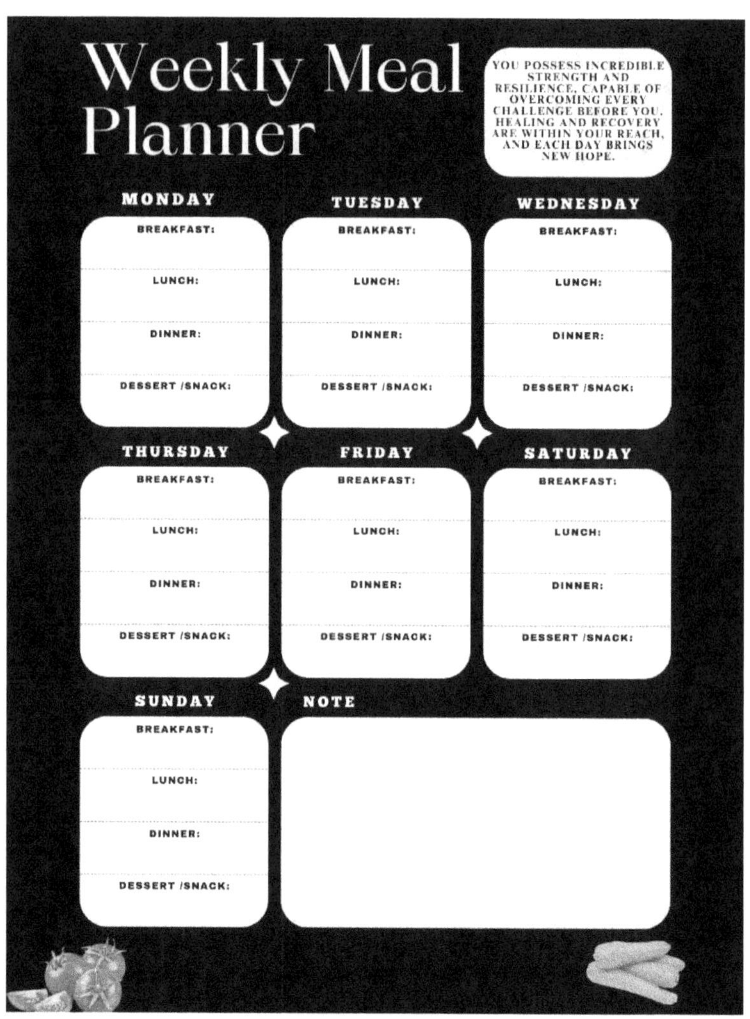

Weekly Meal Planner

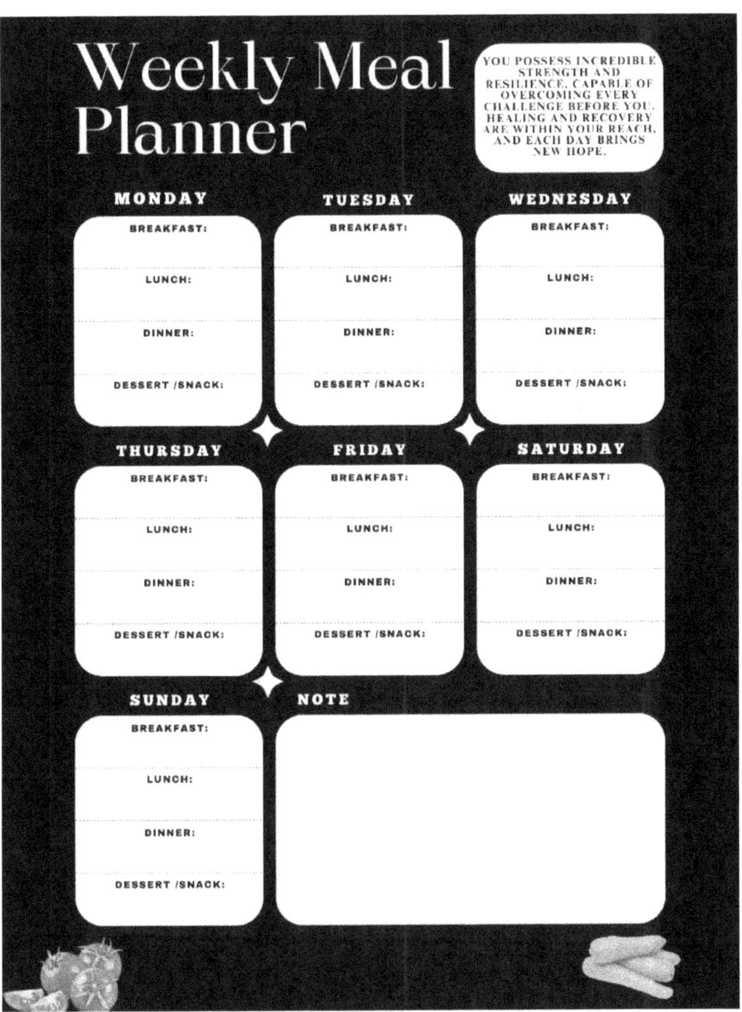

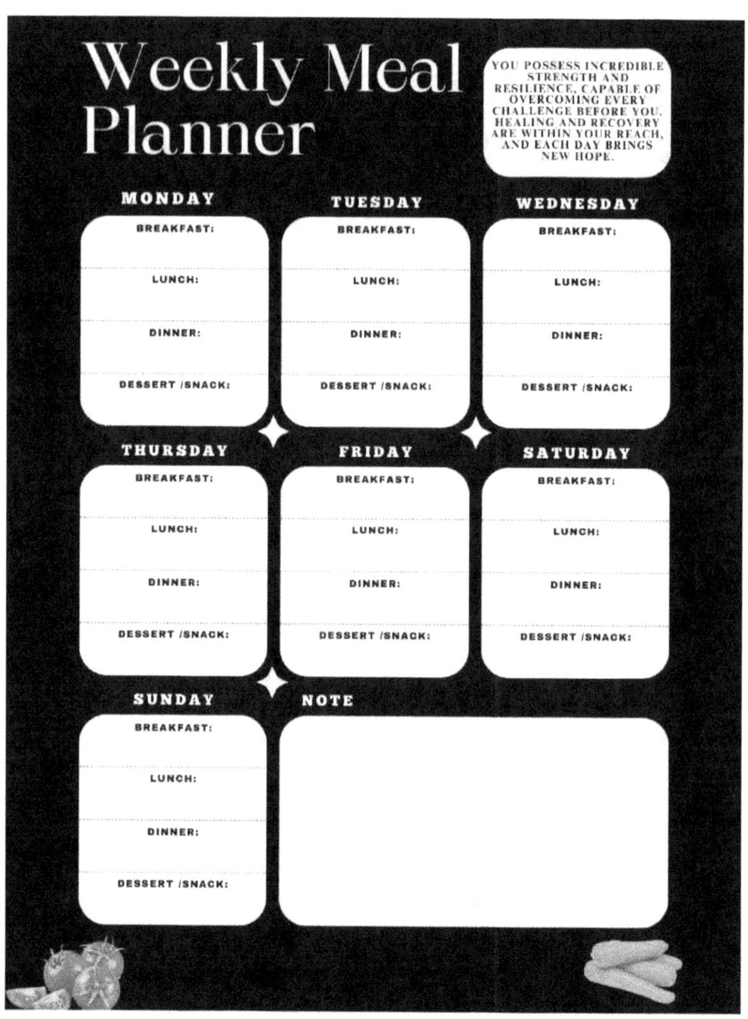

Weekly Meal Planner

YOU POSSESS INCREDIBLE STRENGTH AND RESILIENCE, CAPABLE OF OVERCOMING EVERY CHALLENGE BEFORE YOU. HEALING AND RECOVERY ARE WITHIN YOUR REACH, AND EACH DAY BRINGS NEW HOPE.

MONDAY
BREAKFAST:
LUNCH:
DINNER:
DESSERT /SNACK:

TUESDAY
BREAKFAST:
LUNCH:
DINNER:
DESSERT /SNACK:

WEDNESDAY
BREAKFAST:
LUNCH:
DINNER:
DESSERT /SNACK:

THURSDAY
BREAKFAST:
LUNCH:
DINNER:
DESSERT /SNACK:

FRIDAY
BREAKFAST:
LUNCH:
DINNER:
DESSERT /SNACK:

SATURDAY
BREAKFAST:
LUNCH:
DINNER:
DESSERT /SNACK:

SUNDAY
BREAKFAST:
LUNCH:
DINNER:
DESSERT /SNACK:

NOTE

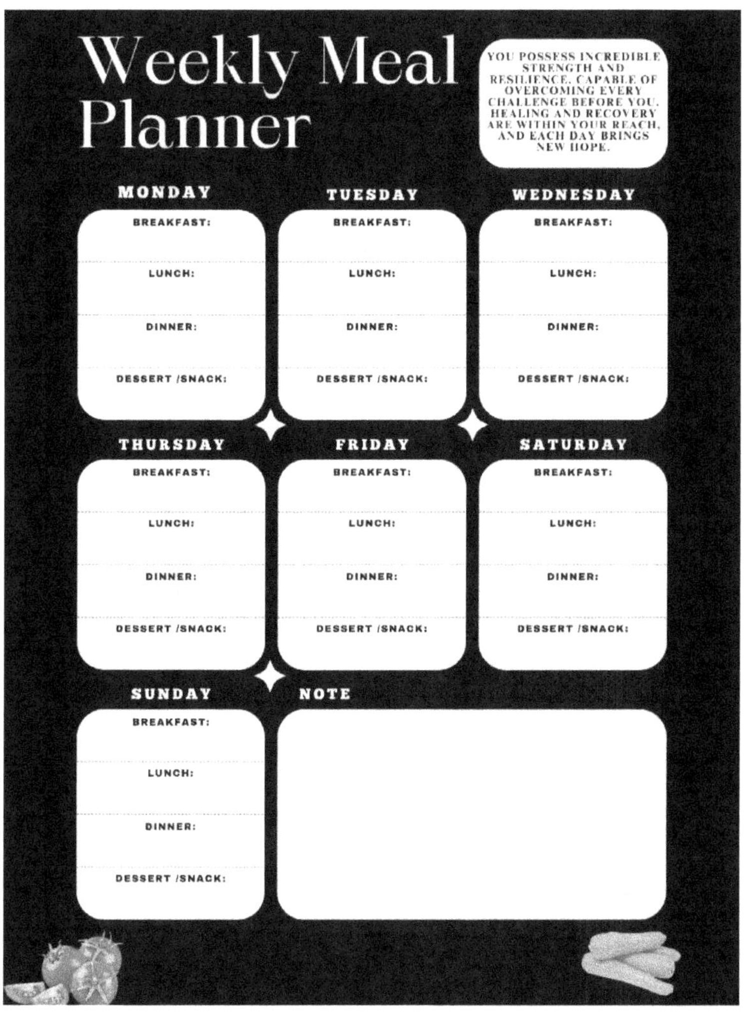

Weekly Meal Planner

YOU POSSESS INCREDIBLE STRENGTH AND RESILIENCE, CAPABLE OF OVERCOMING EVERY CHALLENGE BEFORE YOU. HEALING AND RECOVERY ARE WITHIN YOUR REACH, AND EACH DAY BRINGS NEW HOPE.

MONDAY
BREAKFAST:
LUNCH:
DINNER:
DESSERT /SNACK:

TUESDAY
BREAKFAST:
LUNCH:
DINNER:
DESSERT /SNACK:

WEDNESDAY
BREAKFAST:
LUNCH:
DINNER:
DESSERT /SNACK:

THURSDAY
BREAKFAST:
LUNCH:
DINNER:
DESSERT /SNACK:

FRIDAY
BREAKFAST:
LUNCH:
DINNER:
DESSERT /SNACK:

SATURDAY
BREAKFAST:
LUNCH:
DINNER:
DESSERT /SNACK:

SUNDAY
BREAKFAST:
LUNCH:
DINNER:
DESSERT /SNACK:

NOTE

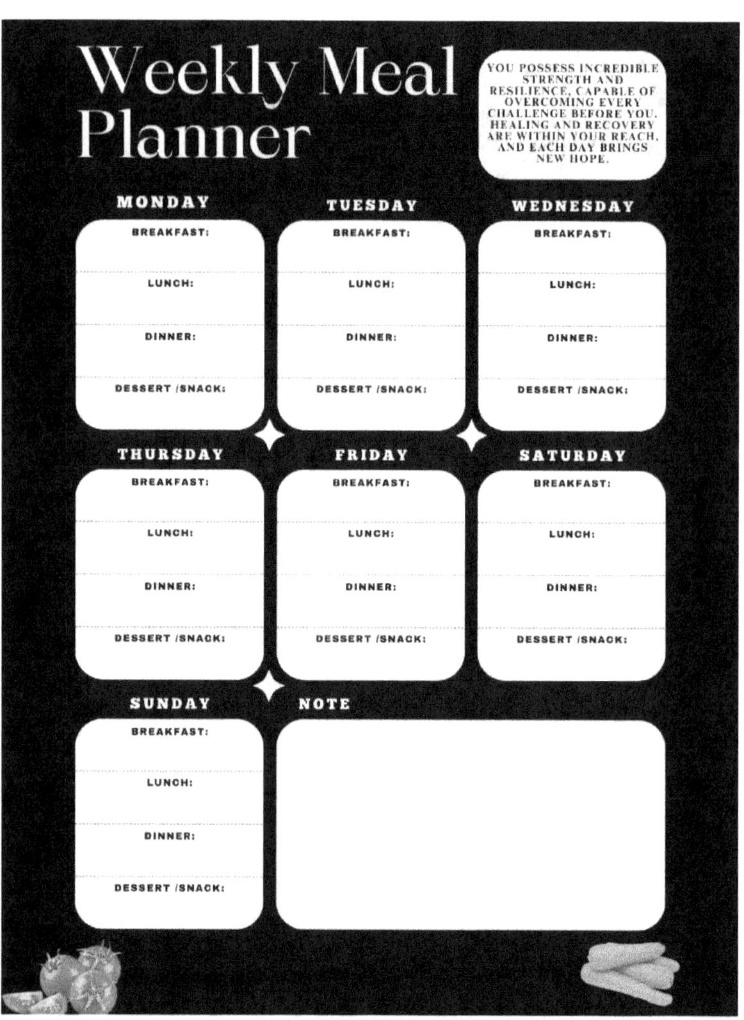

Weekly Meal Planner

YOU POSSESS INCREDIBLE STRENGTH AND RESILIENCE, CAPABLE OF OVERCOMING EVERY CHALLENGE BEFORE YOU. HEALING AND RECOVERY ARE WITHIN YOUR REACH, AND EACH DAY BRINGS NEW HOPE.

MONDAY
BREAKFAST:
LUNCH:
DINNER:
DESSERT /SNACK:

TUESDAY
BREAKFAST:
LUNCH:
DINNER:
DESSERT /SNACK:

WEDNESDAY
BREAKFAST:
LUNCH:
DINNER:
DESSERT /SNACK:

THURSDAY
BREAKFAST:
LUNCH:
DINNER:
DESSERT /SNACK:

FRIDAY
BREAKFAST:
LUNCH:
DINNER:
DESSERT /SNACK:

SATURDAY
BREAKFAST:
LUNCH:
DINNER:
DESSERT /SNACK:

SUNDAY
BREAKFAST:
LUNCH:
DINNER:
DESSERT /SNACK:

NOTE

Weekly Meal Planner

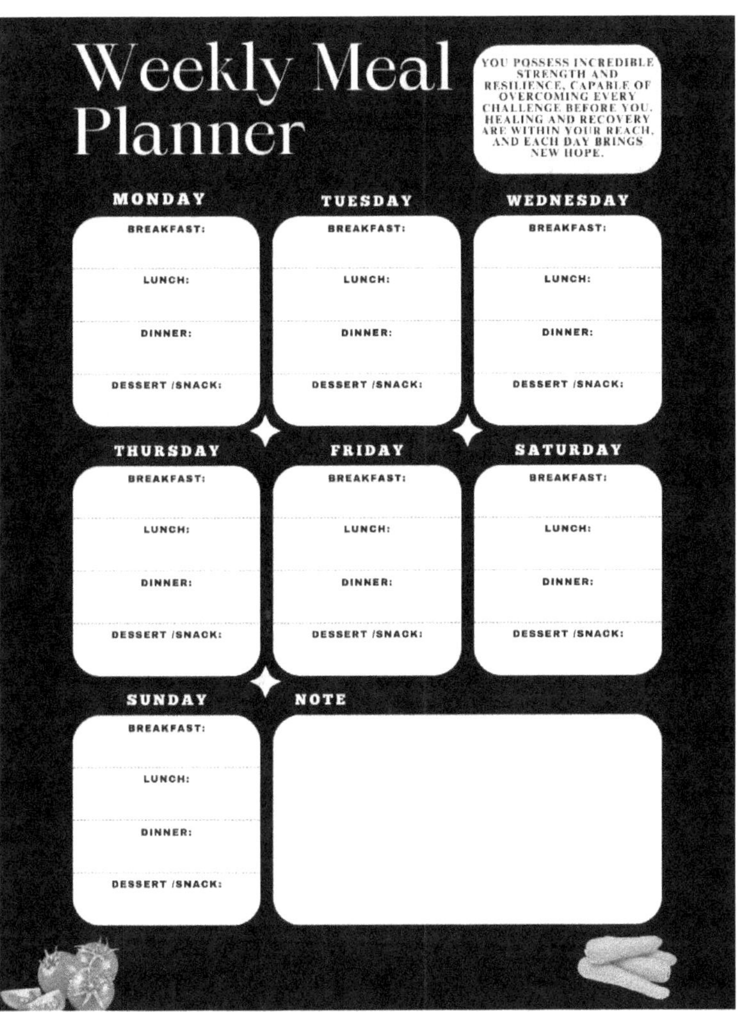

MONDAY
BREAKFAST:
LUNCH:
DINNER:
DESSERT /SNACK:

TUESDAY
BREAKFAST:
LUNCH:
DINNER:
DESSERT /SNACK:

WEDNESDAY
BREAKFAST:
LUNCH:
DINNER:
DESSERT /SNACK:

THURSDAY
BREAKFAST:
LUNCH:
DINNER:
DESSERT /SNACK:

FRIDAY
BREAKFAST:
LUNCH:
DINNER:
DESSERT /SNACK:

SATURDAY
BREAKFAST:
LUNCH:
DINNER:
DESSERT /SNACK:

SUNDAY
BREAKFAST:
LUNCH:
DINNER:
DESSERT /SNACK:

NOTE

Weekly Meal Planner

YOU POSSESS INCREDIBLE STRENGTH AND RESILIENCE, CAPABLE OF OVERCOMING EVERY CHALLENGE BEFORE YOU. HEALING AND RECOVERY ARE WITHIN YOUR REACH, AND EACH DAY BRINGS NEW HOPE.

MONDAY

BREAKFAST:

LUNCH:

DINNER:

DESSERT /SNACK:

TUESDAY

BREAKFAST:

LUNCH:

DINNER:

DESSERT /SNACK:

WEDNESDAY

BREAKFAST:

LUNCH:

DINNER:

DESSERT /SNACK:

THURSDAY

BREAKFAST:

LUNCH:

DINNER:

DESSERT /SNACK:

FRIDAY

BREAKFAST:

LUNCH:

DINNER:

DESSERT /SNACK:

SATURDAY

BREAKFAST:

LUNCH:

DINNER:

DESSERT /SNACK:

SUNDAY

BREAKFAST:

LUNCH:

DINNER:

DESSERT /SNACK:

NOTE

Weekly Meal Planner

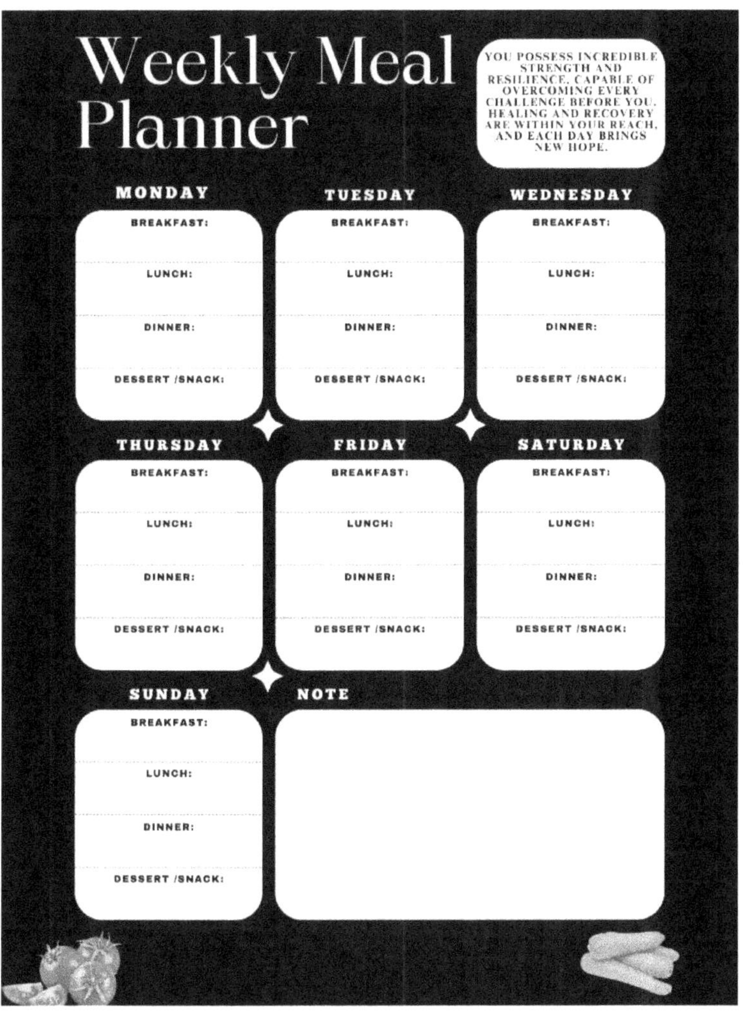

MONDAY

BREAKFAST:

LUNCH:

DINNER:

DESSERT /SNACK:

TUESDAY

BREAKFAST:

LUNCH:

DINNER:

DESSERT /SNACK:

WEDNESDAY

BREAKFAST:

LUNCH:

DINNER:

DESSERT /SNACK:

THURSDAY

BREAKFAST:

LUNCH:

DINNER:

DESSERT /SNACK:

FRIDAY

BREAKFAST:

LUNCH:

DINNER:

DESSERT /SNACK:

SATURDAY

BREAKFAST:

LUNCH:

DINNER:

DESSERT /SNACK:

SUNDAY

BREAKFAST:

LUNCH:

DINNER:

DESSERT /SNACK:

NOTE

Weekly Meal Planner

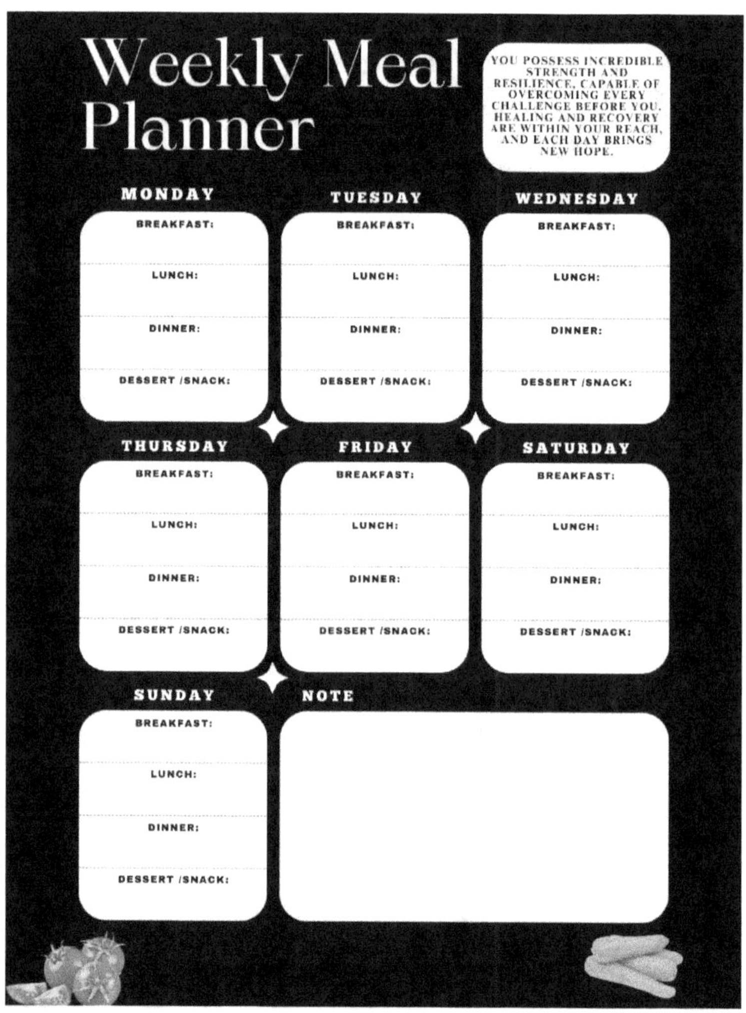

Weekly Meal Planner

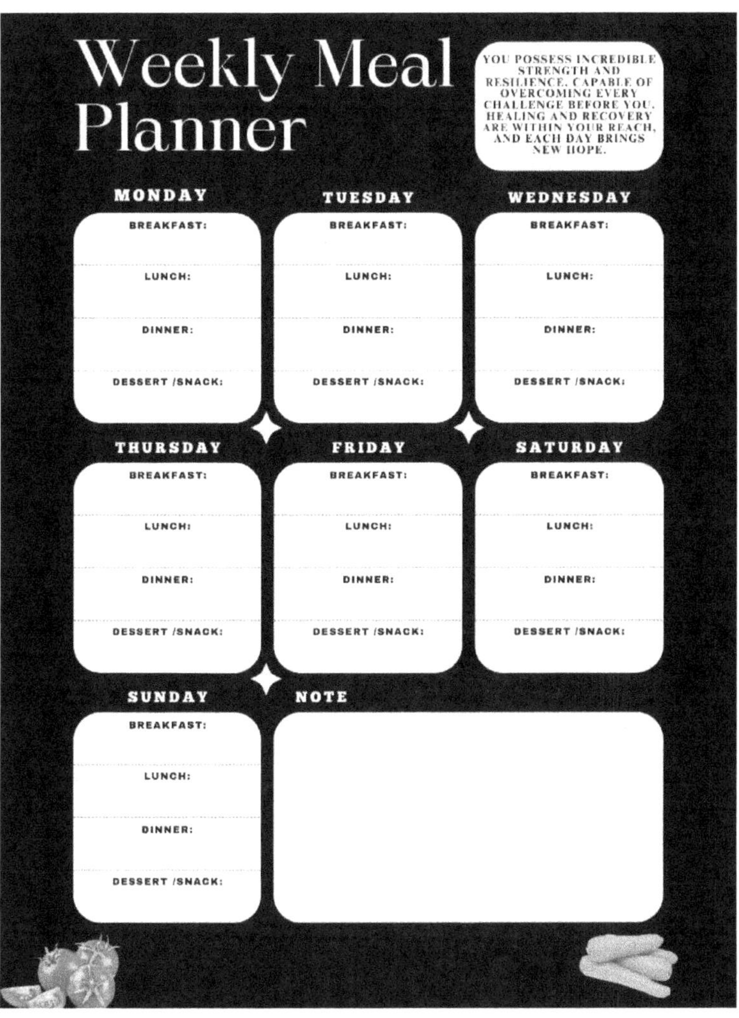

YOU POSSESS INCREDIBLE STRENGTH AND RESILIENCE, CAPABLE OF OVERCOMING EVERY CHALLENGE BEFORE YOU. HEALING AND RECOVERY ARE WITHIN YOUR REACH, AND EACH DAY BRINGS NEW HOPE.

MONDAY

BREAKFAST:

LUNCH:

DINNER:

DESSERT /SNACK:

TUESDAY

BREAKFAST:

LUNCH:

DINNER:

DESSERT /SNACK:

WEDNESDAY

BREAKFAST:

LUNCH:

DINNER:

DESSERT /SNACK:

THURSDAY

BREAKFAST:

LUNCH:

DINNER:

DESSERT /SNACK:

FRIDAY

BREAKFAST:

LUNCH:

DINNER:

DESSERT /SNACK:

SATURDAY

BREAKFAST:

LUNCH:

DINNER:

DESSERT /SNACK:

SUNDAY

BREAKFAST:

LUNCH:

DINNER:

DESSERT /SNACK:

NOTE

Weekly Meal Planner

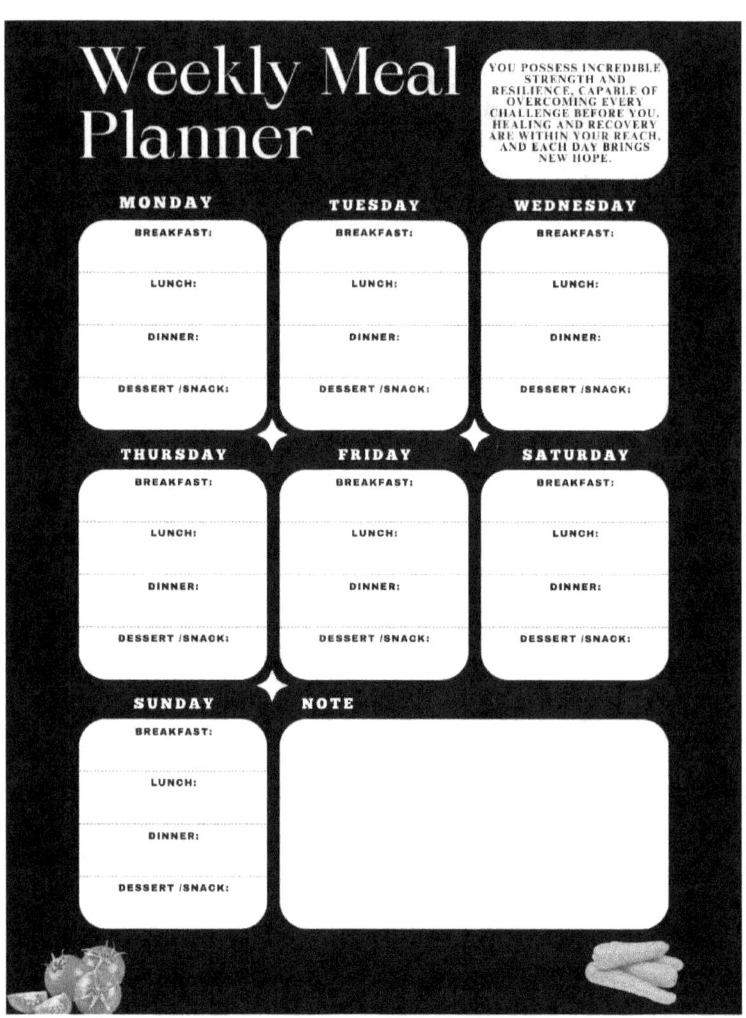

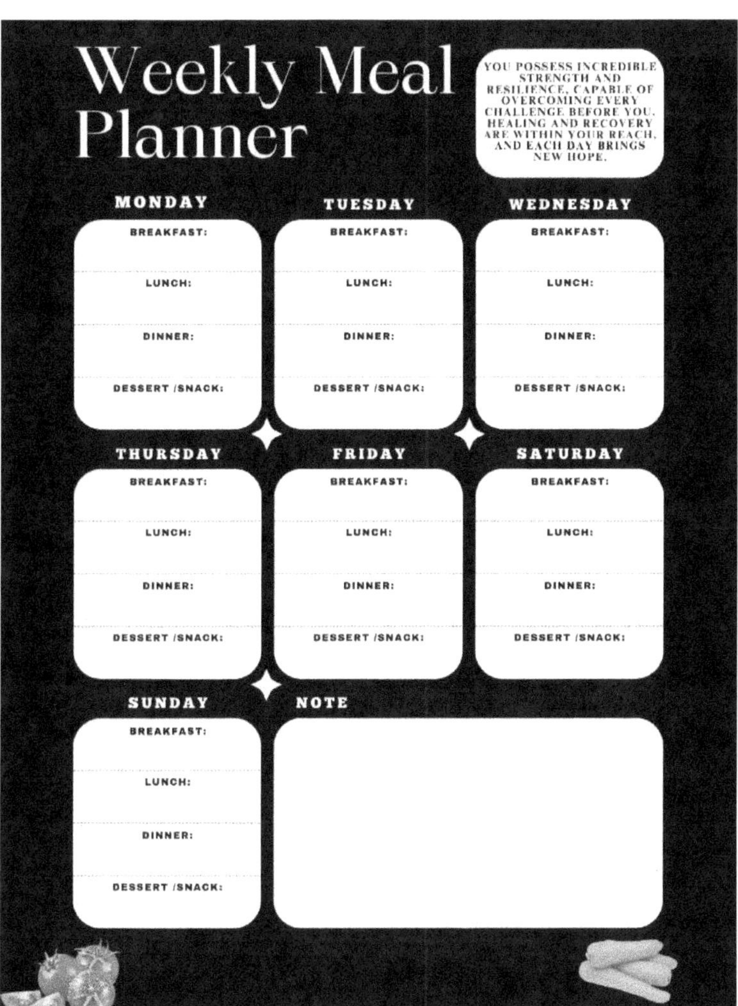

Weekly Meal Planner

YOU POSSESS INCREDIBLE STRENGTH AND RESILIENCE, CAPABLE OF OVERCOMING EVERY CHALLENGE BEFORE YOU. HEALING AND RECOVERY ARE WITHIN YOUR REACH, AND EACH DAY BRINGS NEW HOPE.

MONDAY
BREAKFAST:
LUNCH:
DINNER:
DESSERT /SNACK:

TUESDAY
BREAKFAST:
LUNCH:
DINNER:
DESSERT /SNACK:

WEDNESDAY
BREAKFAST:
LUNCH:
DINNER:
DESSERT /SNACK:

THURSDAY
BREAKFAST:
LUNCH:
DINNER:
DESSERT /SNACK:

FRIDAY
BREAKFAST:
LUNCH:
DINNER:
DESSERT /SNACK:

SATURDAY
BREAKFAST:
LUNCH:
DINNER:
DESSERT /SNACK:

SUNDAY
BREAKFAST:
LUNCH:
DINNER:
DESSERT /SNACK:

NOTE

Weekly Meal Planner

YOU POSSESS INCREDIBLE STRENGTH AND RESILIENCE, CAPABLE OF OVERCOMING EVERY CHALLENGE BEFORE YOU. HEALING AND RECOVERY ARE WITHIN YOUR REACH, AND EACH DAY BRINGS NEW HOPE.

MONDAY

BREAKFAST:

LUNCH:

DINNER:

DESSERT /SNACK:

TUESDAY

BREAKFAST:

LUNCH:

DINNER:

DESSERT /SNACK:

WEDNESDAY

BREAKFAST:

LUNCH:

DINNER:

DESSERT /SNACK:

THURSDAY

BREAKFAST:

LUNCH:

DINNER:

DESSERT /SNACK:

FRIDAY

BREAKFAST:

LUNCH:

DINNER:

DESSERT /SNACK:

SATURDAY

BREAKFAST:

LUNCH:

DINNER:

DESSERT /SNACK:

SUNDAY

BREAKFAST:

LUNCH:

DINNER:

DESSERT /SNACK:

NOTE

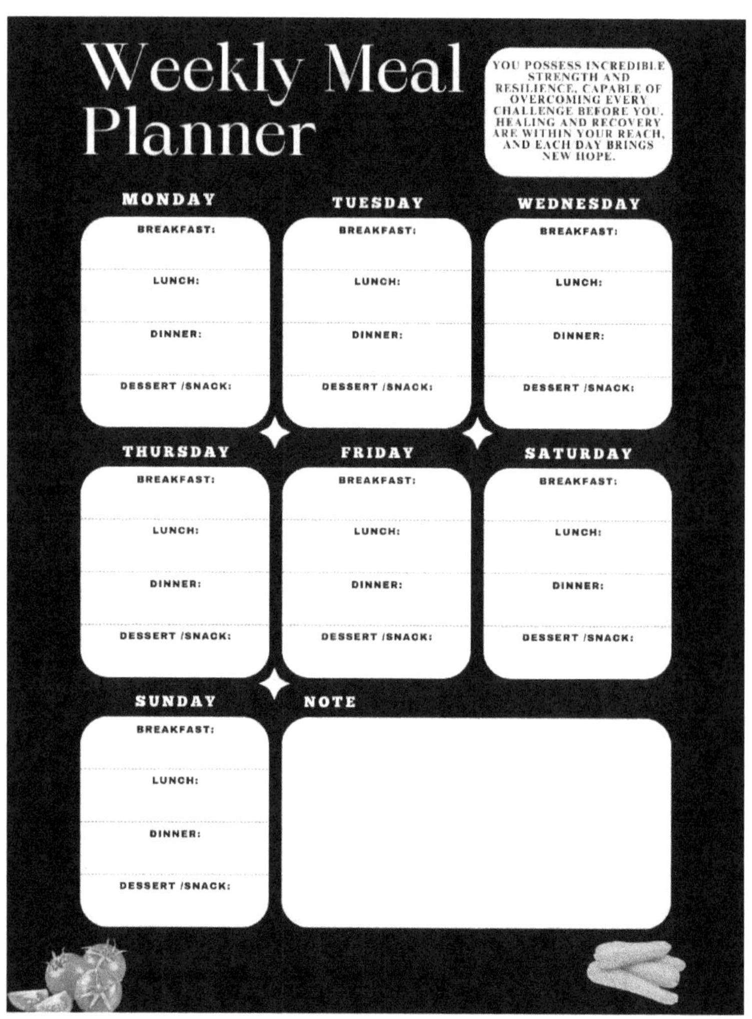

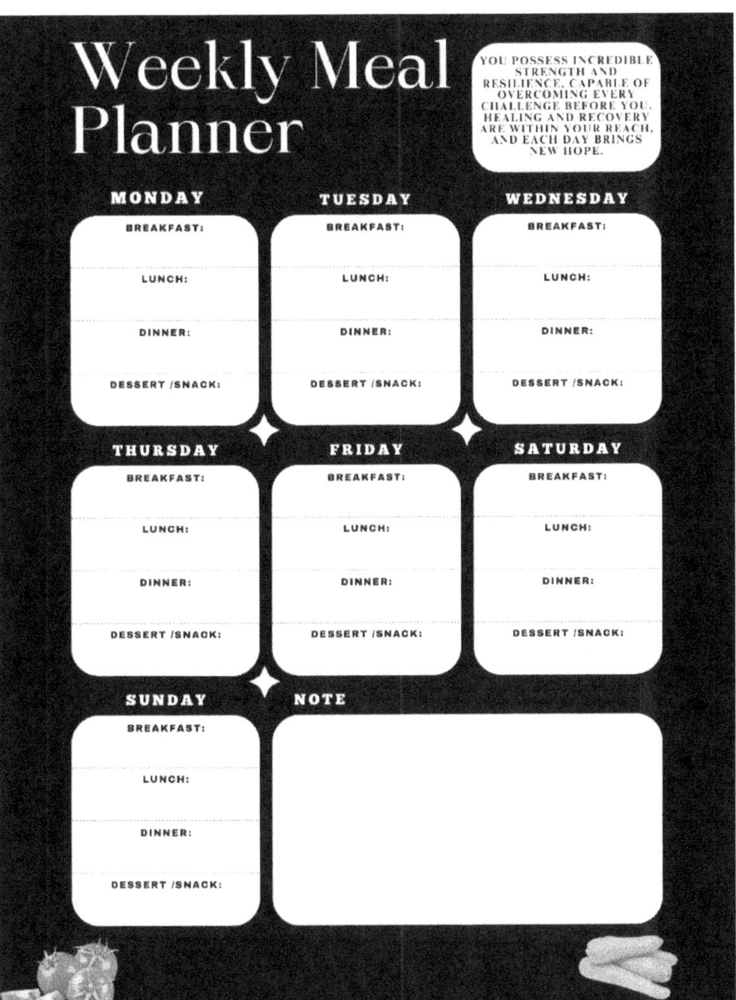

Weekly Meal Planner

YOU POSSESS INCREDIBLE STRENGTH AND RESILIENCE, CAPABLE OF OVERCOMING EVERY CHALLENGE BEFORE YOU. HEALING AND RECOVERY ARE WITHIN YOUR REACH, AND EACH DAY BRINGS NEW HOPE.

MONDAY
BREAKFAST:
LUNCH:
DINNER:
DESSERT /SNACK:

TUESDAY
BREAKFAST:
LUNCH:
DINNER:
DESSERT /SNACK:

WEDNESDAY
BREAKFAST:
LUNCH:
DINNER:
DESSERT /SNACK:

THURSDAY
BREAKFAST:
LUNCH:
DINNER:
DESSERT /SNACK:

FRIDAY
BREAKFAST:
LUNCH:
DINNER:
DESSERT /SNACK:

SATURDAY
BREAKFAST:
LUNCH:
DINNER:
DESSERT /SNACK:

SUNDAY
BREAKFAST:
LUNCH:
DINNER:
DESSERT /SNACK:

NOTE

Weekly Meal Planner

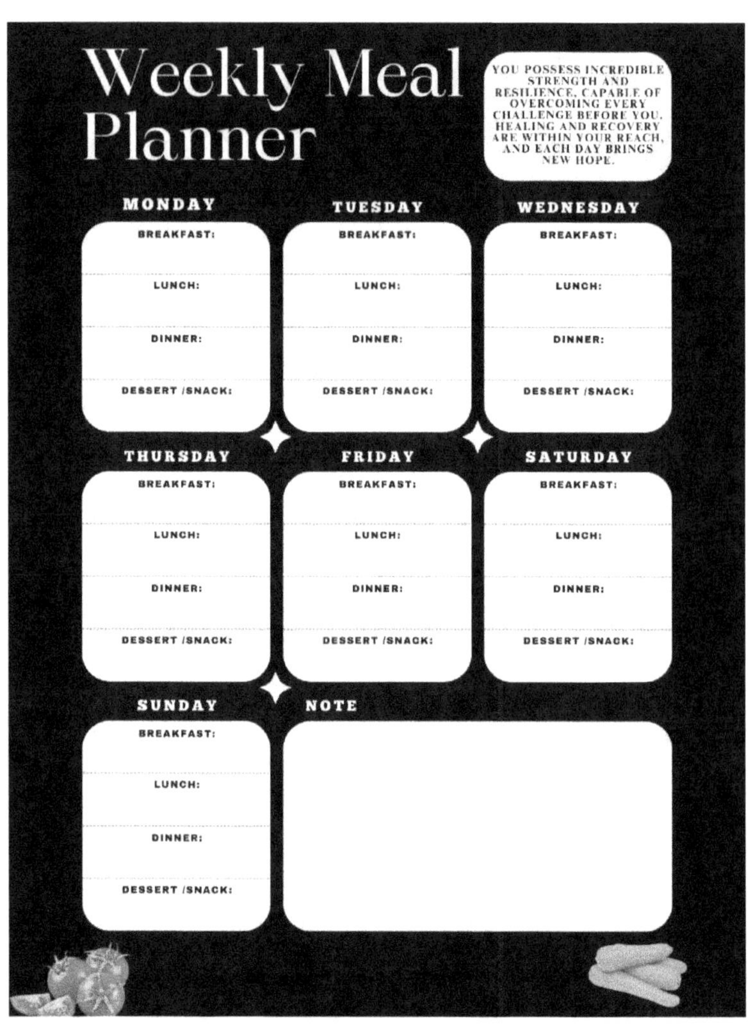

Weekly Meal Planner

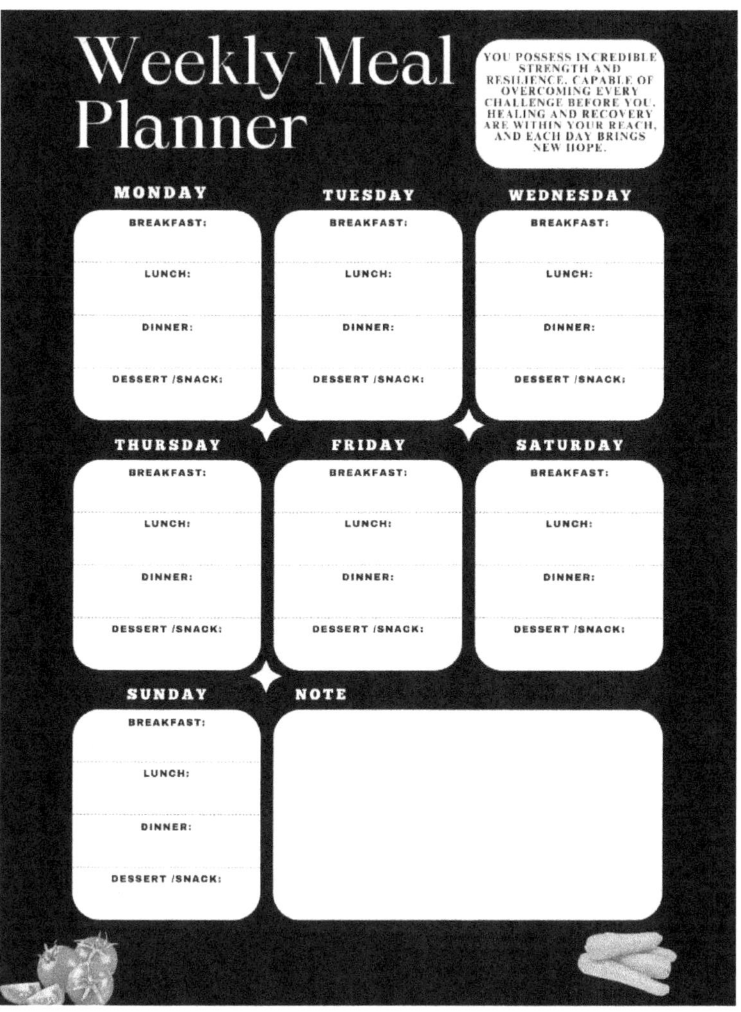

MONDAY
BREAKFAST:

LUNCH:

DINNER:

DESSERT /SNACK:

TUESDAY
BREAKFAST:

LUNCH:

DINNER:

DESSERT /SNACK:

WEDNESDAY
BREAKFAST:

LUNCH:

DINNER:

DESSERT /SNACK:

THURSDAY
BREAKFAST:

LUNCH:

DINNER:

DESSERT /SNACK:

FRIDAY
BREAKFAST:

LUNCH:

DINNER:

DESSERT /SNACK:

SATURDAY
BREAKFAST:

LUNCH:

DINNER:

DESSERT /SNACK:

SUNDAY
BREAKFAST:

LUNCH:

DINNER:

DESSERT /SNACK:

NOTE

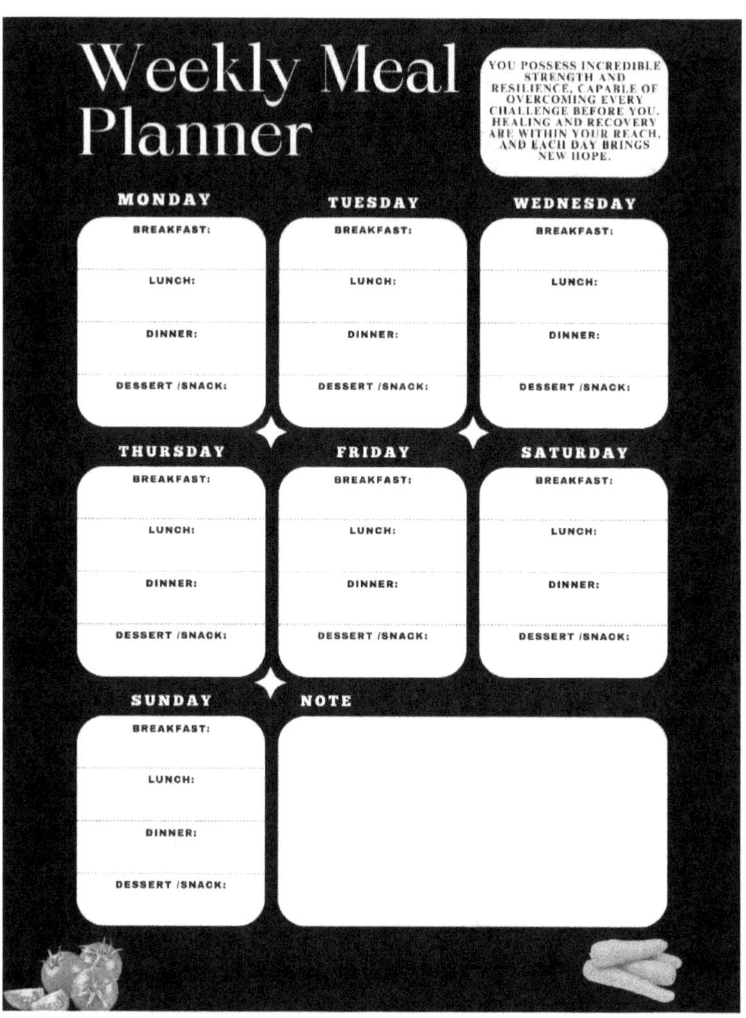

Weekly Meal Planner
YOU POSSESS INCREDIBLE STRENGTH AND RESILIENCE, CAPABLE OF OVERCOMING EVERY CHALLENGE BEFORE YOU. HEALING AND RECOVERY ARE WITHIN YOUR REACH, AND EACH DAY BRINGS NEW HOPE.
MONDAY
BREAKFAST:
LUNCH:
DINNER:
DESSERT /SNACK:
TUESDAY
BREAKFAST:
LUNCH:
DINNER:
DESSERT /SNACK:
WEDNESDAY
BREAKFAST:
LUNCH:
DINNER:
DESSERT /SNACK:
THURSDAY
BREAKFAST:
LUNCH:
DINNER:
DESSERT /SNACK:
FRIDAY
BREAKFAST:
LUNCH:
DINNER:
DESSERT /SNACK:
SATURDAY
BREAKFAST:
LUNCH:
DINNER:
DESSERT /SNACK:
SUNDAY
BREAKFAST:
LUNCH:
DINNER:
DESSERT /SNACK:
NOTE

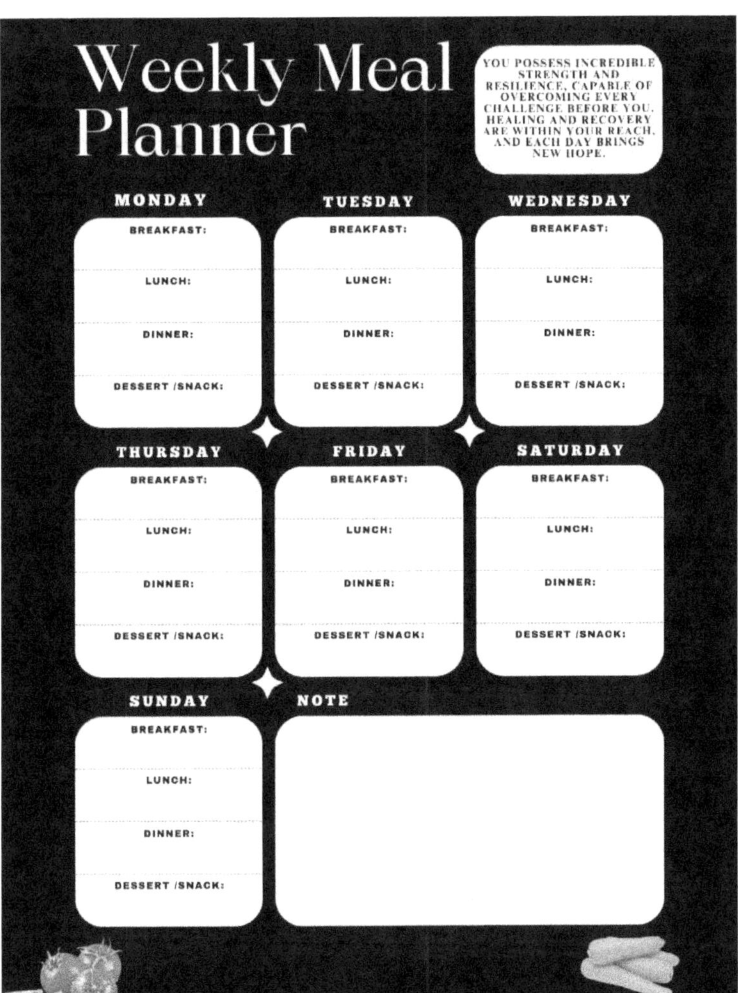

Weekly Meal Planner

YOU POSSESS INCREDIBLE STRENGTH AND RESILIENCE, CAPABLE OF OVERCOMING EVERY CHALLENGE BEFORE YOU. HEALING AND RECOVERY ARE WITHIN YOUR REACH, AND EACH DAY BRINGS NEW HOPE.

MONDAY
BREAKFAST:
LUNCH:
DINNER:
DESSERT /SNACK:

TUESDAY
BREAKFAST:
LUNCH:
DINNER:
DESSERT /SNACK:

WEDNESDAY
BREAKFAST:
LUNCH:
DINNER:
DESSERT /SNACK:

THURSDAY
BREAKFAST:
LUNCH:
DINNER:
DESSERT /SNACK:

FRIDAY
BREAKFAST:
LUNCH:
DINNER:
DESSERT /SNACK:

SATURDAY
BREAKFAST:
LUNCH:
DINNER:
DESSERT /SNACK:

SUNDAY
BREAKFAST:
LUNCH:
DINNER:
DESSERT /SNACK:

NOTE

Weekly Meal Planner

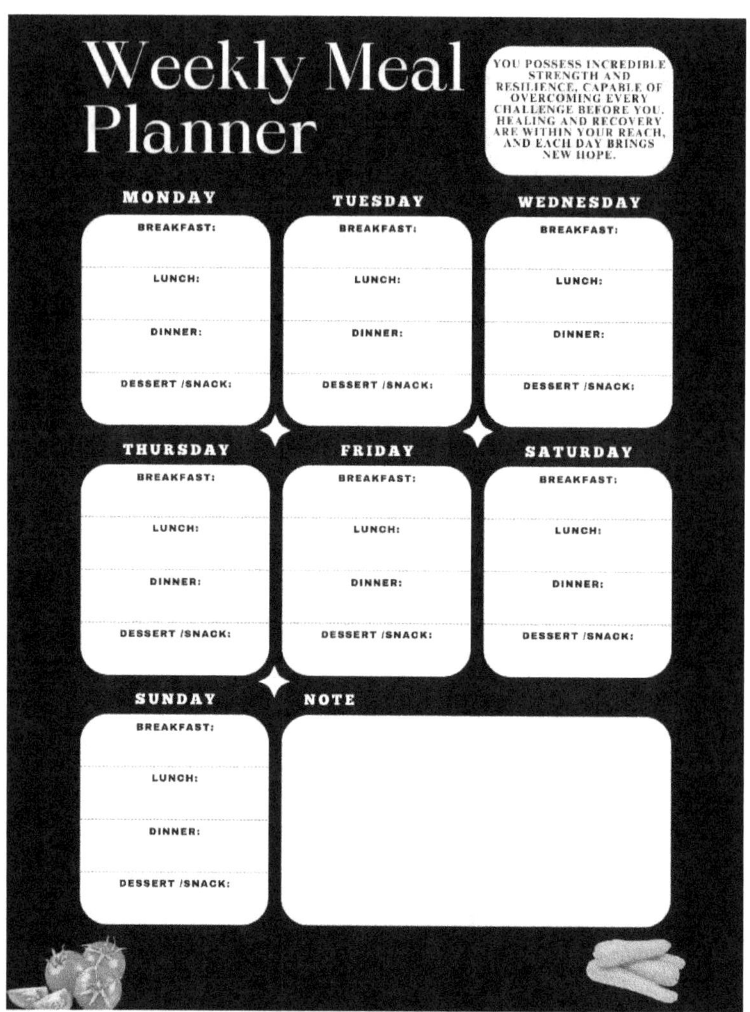

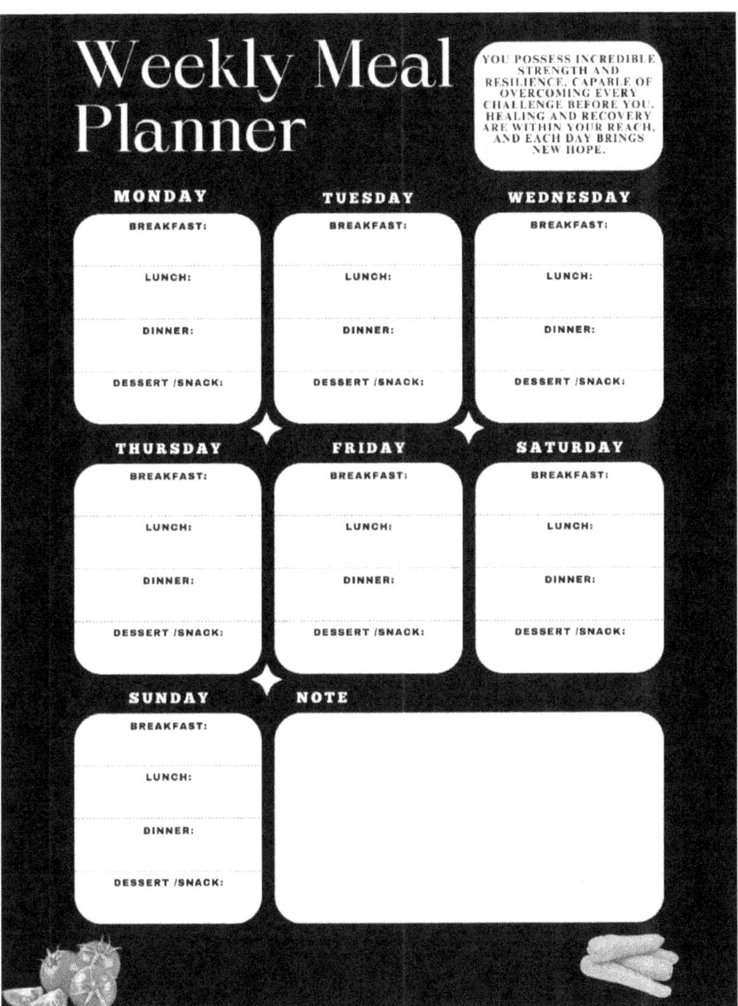

Weekly Meal Planner

YOU POSSESS INCREDIBLE
STRENGTH AND
RESILIENCE, CAPABLE OF
OVERCOMING EVERY
CHALLENGE BEFORE YOU.
HEALING AND RECOVERY
ARE WITHIN YOUR REACH,
AND EACH DAY BRINGS
NEW HOPE.

MONDAY
BREAKFAST:
LUNCH:
DINNER:
DESSERT /SNACK:

TUESDAY
BREAKFAST:
LUNCH:
DINNER:
DESSERT /SNACK:

WEDNESDAY
BREAKFAST:
LUNCH:
DINNER:
DESSERT /SNACK:

THURSDAY
BREAKFAST:
LUNCH:
DINNER:
DESSERT /SNACK:

FRIDAY
BREAKFAST:
LUNCH:
DINNER:
DESSERT /SNACK:

SATURDAY
BREAKFAST:
LUNCH:
DINNER:
DESSERT /SNACK:

SUNDAY
BREAKFAST:
LUNCH:
DINNER:
DESSERT /SNACK:

NOTE

Weekly Meal Planner

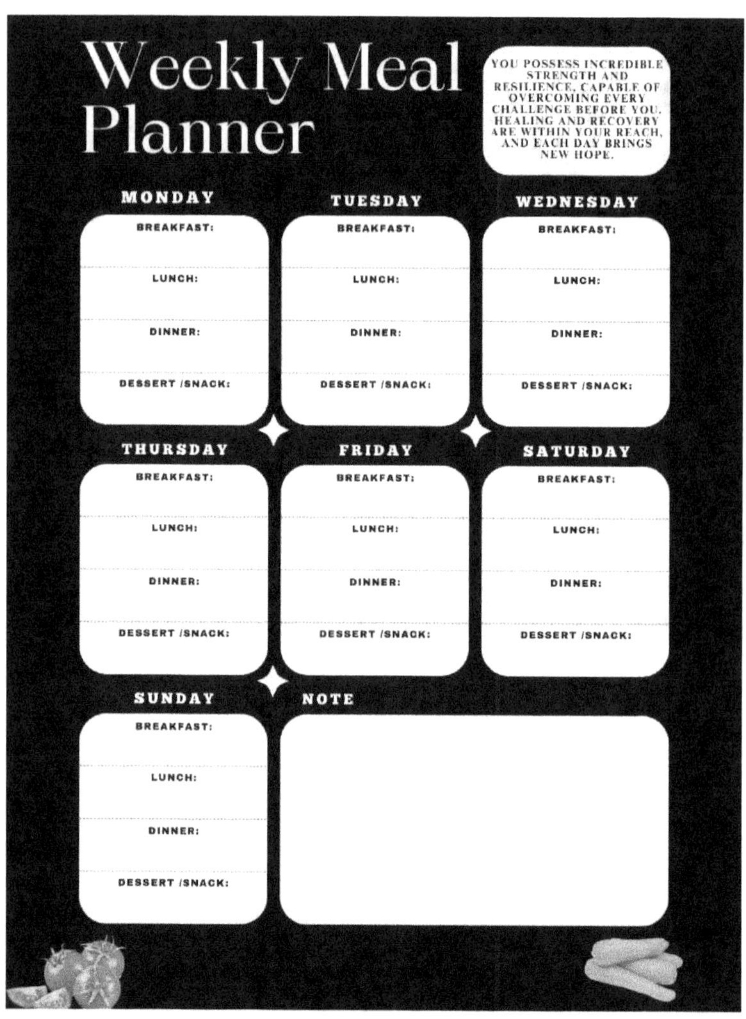

Weekly Meal Planner

YOU POSSESS INCREDIBLE STRENGTH AND RESILIENCE, CAPABLE OF OVERCOMING EVERY CHALLENGE BEFORE YOU. HEALING AND RECOVERY ARE WITHIN YOUR REACH, AND EACH DAY BRINGS NEW HOPE.

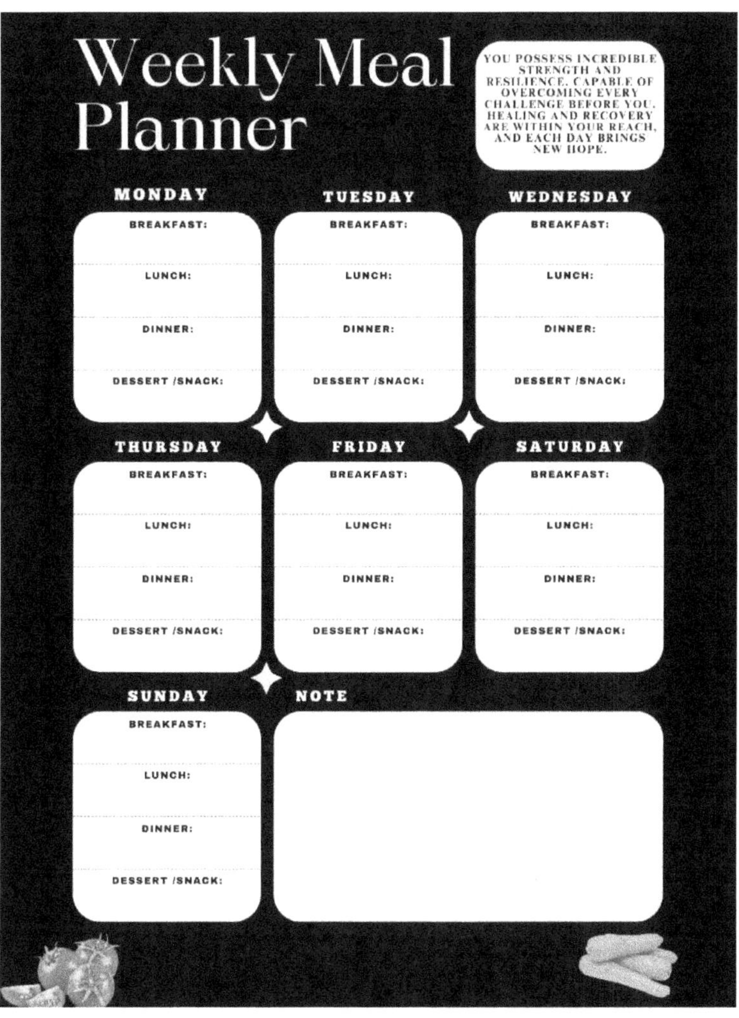

Weekly Meal Planner

> YOU POSSESS INCREDIBLE STRENGTH AND RESILIENCE, CAPABLE OF OVERCOMING EVERY CHALLENGE BEFORE YOU. HEALING AND RECOVERY ARE WITHIN YOUR REACH, AND EACH DAY BRINGS NEW HOPE.

MONDAY
BREAKFAST:

LUNCH:

DINNER:

DESSERT /SNACK:

TUESDAY
BREAKFAST:

LUNCH:

DINNER:

DESSERT /SNACK:

WEDNESDAY
BREAKFAST:

LUNCH:

DINNER:

DESSERT /SNACK:

THURSDAY
BREAKFAST:

LUNCH:

DINNER:

DESSERT /SNACK:

FRIDAY
BREAKFAST:

LUNCH:

DINNER:

DESSERT /SNACK:

SATURDAY
BREAKFAST:

LUNCH:

DINNER:

DESSERT /SNACK:

SUNDAY
BREAKFAST:

LUNCH:

DINNER:

DESSERT /SNACK:

NOTE

Weekly Meal Planner

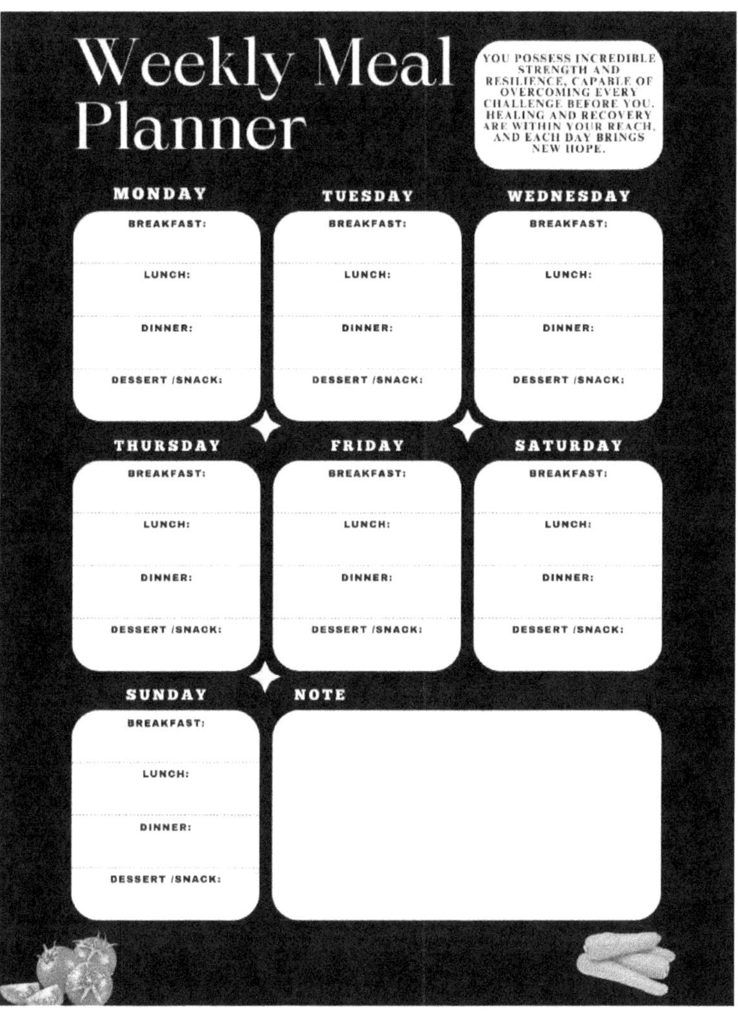

Weekly Meal Planner

YOU POSSESS INCREDIBLE STRENGTH AND RESILIENCE, CAPABLE OF OVERCOMING EVERY CHALLENGE BEFORE YOU. HEALING AND RECOVERY ARE WITHIN YOUR REACH, AND EACH DAY BRINGS NEW HOPE.

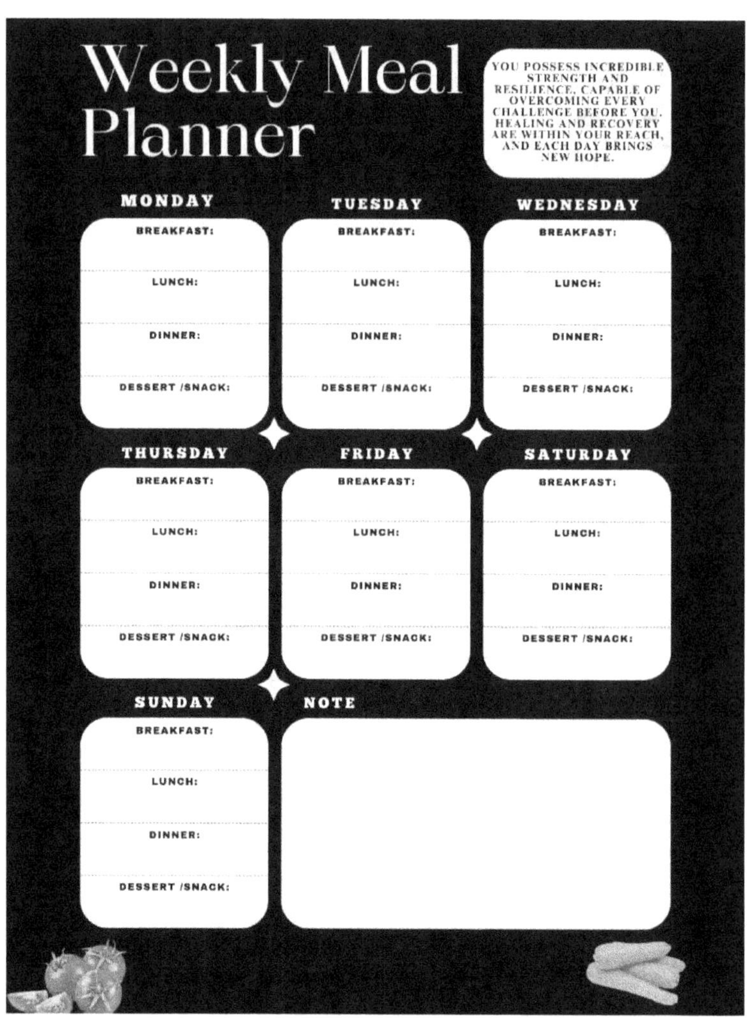

MONDAY

BREAKFAST:

LUNCH:

DINNER:

DESSERT /SNACK:

TUESDAY

BREAKFAST:

LUNCH:

DINNER:

DESSERT /SNACK:

WEDNESDAY

BREAKFAST:

LUNCH:

DINNER:

DESSERT /SNACK:

THURSDAY

BREAKFAST:

LUNCH:

DINNER:

DESSERT /SNACK:

FRIDAY

BREAKFAST:

LUNCH:

DINNER:

DESSERT /SNACK:

SATURDAY

BREAKFAST:

LUNCH:

DINNER:

DESSERT /SNACK:

SUNDAY

BREAKFAST:

LUNCH:

DINNER:

DESSERT /SNACK:

NOTE

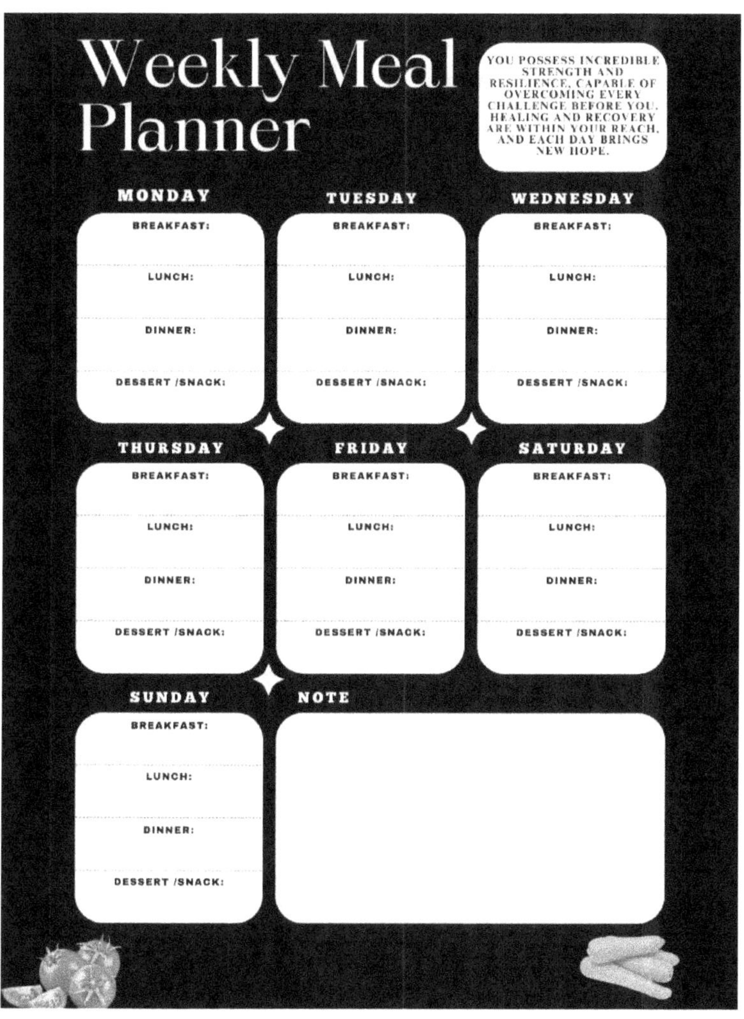

Weekly Meal Planner

YOU POSSESS INCREDIBLE STRENGTH AND RESILIENCE, CAPABLE OF OVERCOMING EVERY CHALLENGE BEFORE YOU. HEALING AND RECOVERY ARE WITHIN YOUR REACH, AND EACH DAY BRINGS NEW HOPE.

MONDAY
BREAKFAST:
LUNCH:
DINNER:
DESSERT /SNACK:

TUESDAY
BREAKFAST:
LUNCH:
DINNER:
DESSERT /SNACK:

WEDNESDAY
BREAKFAST:
LUNCH:
DINNER:
DESSERT /SNACK:

THURSDAY
BREAKFAST:
LUNCH:
DINNER:
DESSERT /SNACK:

FRIDAY
BREAKFAST:
LUNCH:
DINNER:
DESSERT /SNACK:

SATURDAY
BREAKFAST:
LUNCH:
DINNER:
DESSERT /SNACK:

SUNDAY
BREAKFAST:
LUNCH:
DINNER:
DESSERT /SNACK:

NOTE

Weekly Meal Planner

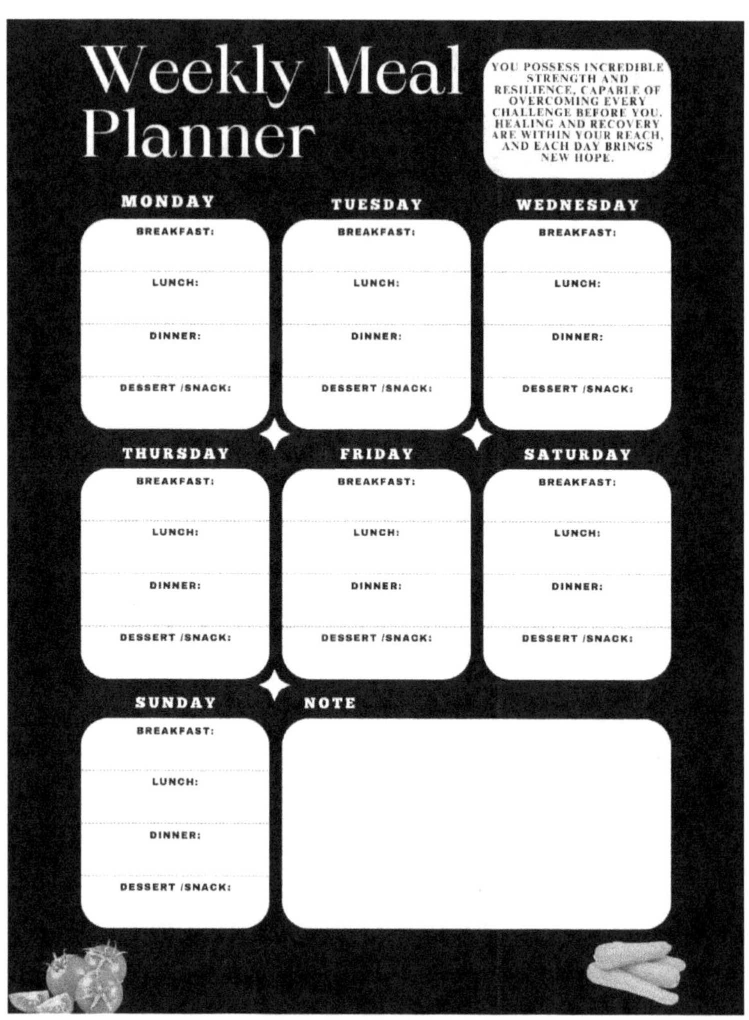

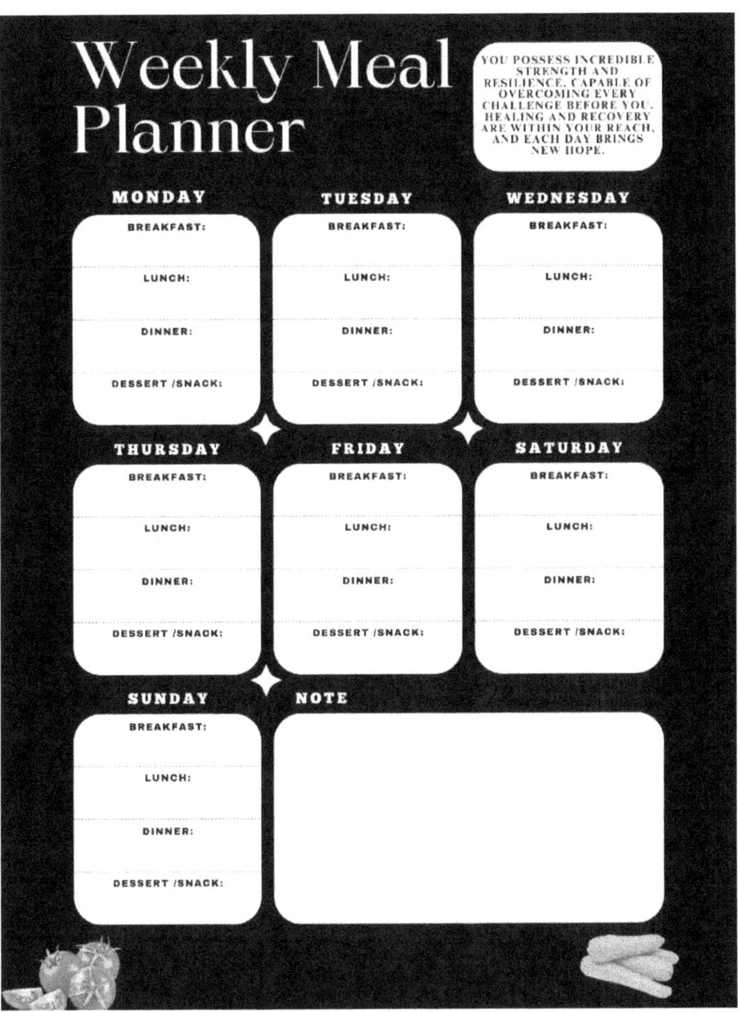

Weekly Meal Planner

YOU POSSESS INCREDIBLE STRENGTH AND RESILIENCE, CAPABLE OF OVERCOMING EVERY CHALLENGE BEFORE YOU. HEALING AND RECOVERY ARE WITHIN YOUR REACH, AND EACH DAY BRINGS NEW HOPE.

MONDAY
BREAKFAST:
LUNCH:
DINNER:
DESSERT /SNACK:

TUESDAY
BREAKFAST:
LUNCH:
DINNER:
DESSERT /SNACK:

WEDNESDAY
BREAKFAST:
LUNCH:
DINNER:
DESSERT /SNACK:

THURSDAY
BREAKFAST:
LUNCH:
DINNER:
DESSERT /SNACK:

FRIDAY
BREAKFAST:
LUNCH:
DINNER:
DESSERT /SNACK:

SATURDAY
BREAKFAST:
LUNCH:
DINNER:
DESSERT /SNACK:

SUNDAY
BREAKFAST:
LUNCH:
DINNER:
DESSERT /SNACK:

NOTE

Weekly Meal Planner

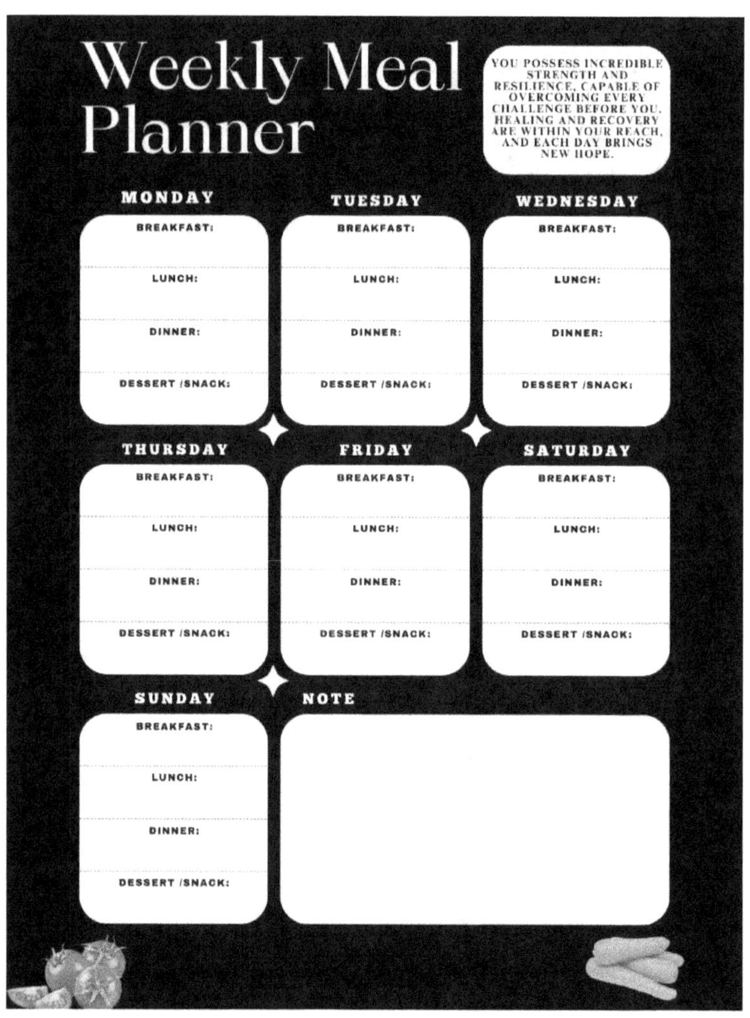

Weekly Meal Planner

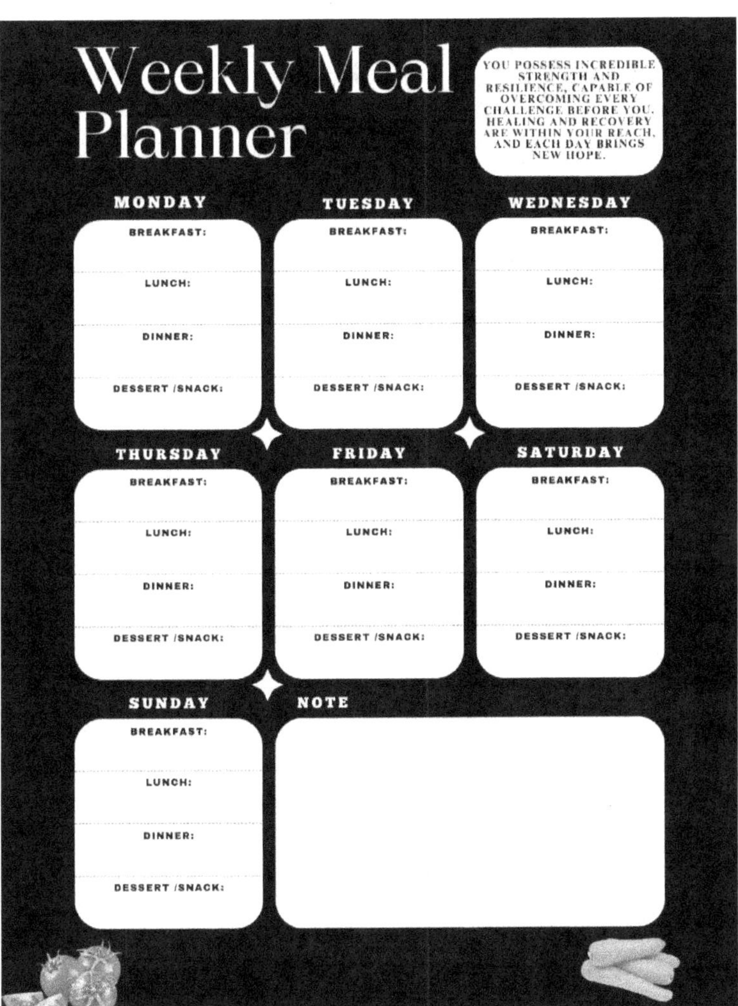

Weekly Meal Planner

YOU POSSESS INCREDIBLE STRENGTH AND RESILIENCE, CAPABLE OF OVERCOMING EVERY CHALLENGE BEFORE YOU. HEALING AND RECOVERY ARE WITHIN YOUR REACH, AND EACH DAY BRINGS NEW HOPE.

MONDAY
BREAKFAST:

LUNCH:

DINNER:

DESSERT /SNACK:

TUESDAY
BREAKFAST:

LUNCH:

DINNER:

DESSERT /SNACK:

WEDNESDAY
BREAKFAST:

LUNCH:

DINNER:

DESSERT /SNACK:

THURSDAY
BREAKFAST:

LUNCH:

DINNER:

DESSERT /SNACK:

FRIDAY
BREAKFAST:

LUNCH:

DINNER:

DESSERT /SNACK:

SATURDAY
BREAKFAST:

LUNCH:

DINNER:

DESSERT /SNACK:

SUNDAY
BREAKFAST:

LUNCH:

DINNER:

DESSERT /SNACK:

NOTE

Weekly Meal Planner

> YOU POSSESS INCREDIBLE STRENGTH AND RESILIENCE, CAPABLE OF OVERCOMING EVERY CHALLENGE BEFORE YOU. HEALING AND RECOVERY ARE WITHIN YOUR REACH, AND EACH DAY BRINGS NEW HOPE.

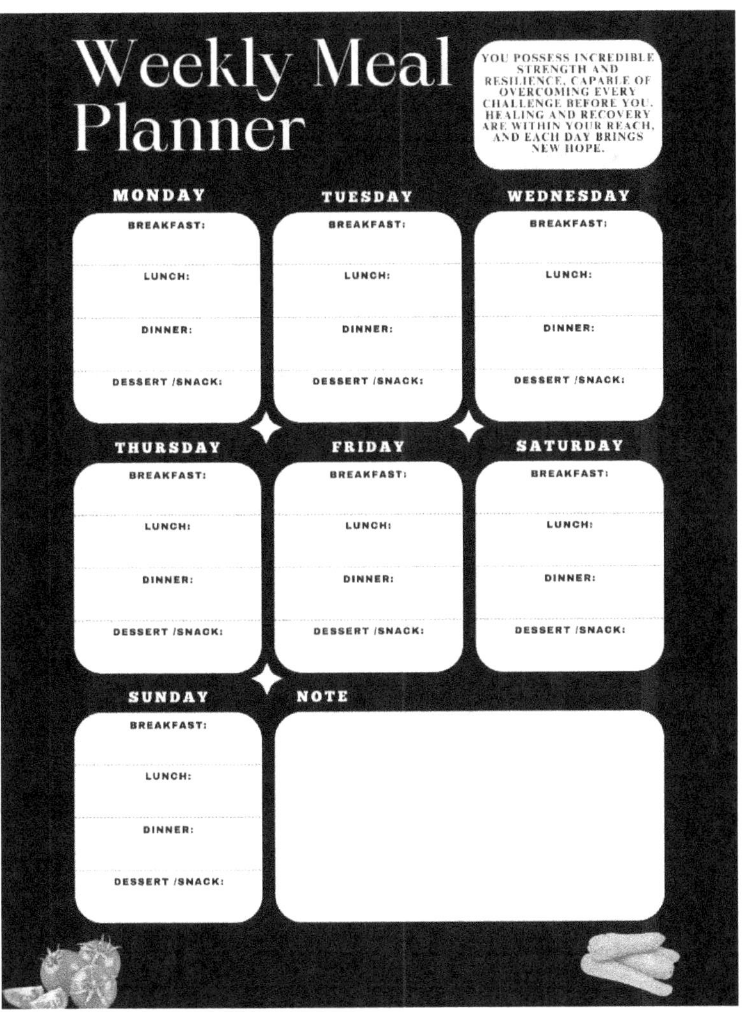

MONDAY
BREAKFAST:

LUNCH:

DINNER:

DESSERT /SNACK:

TUESDAY
BREAKFAST:

LUNCH:

DINNER:

DESSERT /SNACK:

WEDNESDAY
BREAKFAST:

LUNCH:

DINNER:

DESSERT /SNACK:

THURSDAY
BREAKFAST:

LUNCH:

DINNER:

DESSERT /SNACK:

FRIDAY
BREAKFAST:

LUNCH:

DINNER:

DESSERT /SNACK:

SATURDAY
BREAKFAST:

LUNCH:

DINNER:

DESSERT /SNACK:

SUNDAY
BREAKFAST:

LUNCH:

DINNER:

DESSERT /SNACK:

NOTE

Weekly Meal Planner

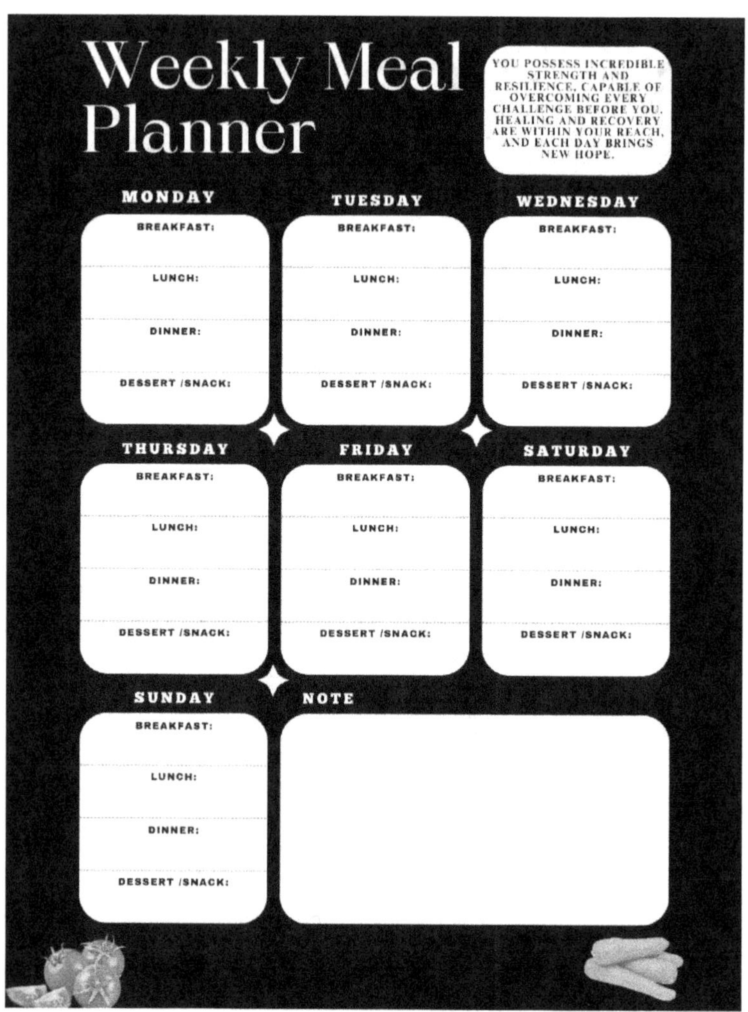

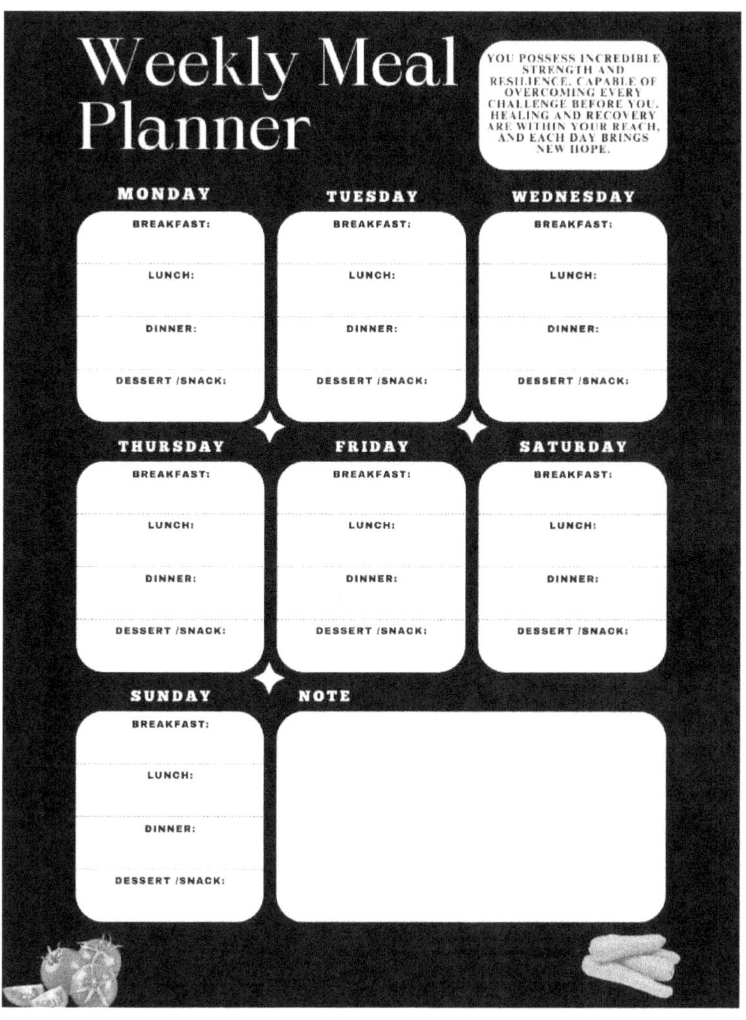

Weekly Meal Planner

YOU POSSESS INCREDIBLE STRENGTH AND RESILIENCE, CAPABLE OF OVERCOMING EVERY CHALLENGE BEFORE YOU. HEALING AND RECOVERY ARE WITHIN YOUR REACH, AND EACH DAY BRINGS NEW HOPE.

MONDAY
BREAKFAST:
LUNCH:
DINNER:
DESSERT /SNACK:

TUESDAY
BREAKFAST:
LUNCH:
DINNER:
DESSERT /SNACK:

WEDNESDAY
BREAKFAST:
LUNCH:
DINNER:
DESSERT /SNACK:

THURSDAY
BREAKFAST:
LUNCH:
DINNER:
DESSERT /SNACK:

FRIDAY
BREAKFAST:
LUNCH:
DINNER:
DESSERT /SNACK:

SATURDAY
BREAKFAST:
LUNCH:
DINNER:
DESSERT /SNACK:

SUNDAY
BREAKFAST:
LUNCH:
DINNER:
DESSERT /SNACK:

NOTE

* 9 7 9 8 3 2 6 2 4 9 4 5 6 *